Radiographic Anatomy, Positioning, and Procedures Workbook

VOLUME TWO

*This workbook is dedicated to the most important person in my life,
my wife, Sharon Hayes. Her love and support for me have created all the happiness
in my life. She was the motivation that inspired me to become
a radiologic technology educator, and she is the reason I still pursue goals;
therefore this publication is for her.*

Radiographic Anatomy, Positioning, and Procedures Workbook

VOLUME TWO

SECOND EDITION

Steven G. Hayes Sr., BSRT, MEd, RT(R)

St. Louis Baltimore Boston Carlsbad Chicago Minneapolis New York Philadelphia Portland
London Milan Sydney Tokyo Toronto

Publisher: Don E. Ladig
Executive Editor: Jeanne Rowland
Developmental Editor: Carole Glauser
Project Manager: Linda McKinley
Production Editor: René Spencer Saller
Design Coordinator: Renée Duenow
Book Design: Graphic World Publishing Services
Cover Design: Acme Creative Studios
Manufacturing Supervisor: Karen Boehme

SECOND EDITION

Mosby, Inc.
11830 Westline Industrial Drive
St. Louis, Missouri 63146
www.mosby.com

International Standard Book Number: 0-323-00229-3

99 00 01 02 03 / 9 8 7 6 5 4 3 2

Reviewers

Joseph Dielman, BS, RT
Radiographer
Hoffman Estates Medical Center
Department of Medical Imaging
Hoffman Estates, Illinois

Ellen Dikun, BS, RT (ARRT)
Instructor
Middlesex County College
Department of Radiography Education
Edison, New Jersey

Kenneth Roszel, MS, RT(R)
Member Education Coordinator
Penn State Geisinger Health System
Bloomsburg, Pennsylvania

Rhonda Stadt Wahl, PhD, RT(R)
Assistant Professor
University of Missouri
Department of Cardiopulmonary and Diagnostic Studies
Columbia, Missouri

Lettie Sutton, BAS, RT(R)
Clinical Coordinator
Radiography Program
Fayetteville Technical Community College
Fayetteville, North Carolina

Andrew Woodward, MA, RT (R)(ARRT)
Department Head/Assistant Professor
Radiologic Technology
WOR-WIC Community College
Salisbury, Maryland

Preface

This two-volume workbook has been developed to accompany *Mosby's Radiographic Instructional Series: Anatomy, Positioning, and Procedures* multimedia and *Merrill's Atlas of Radiographic Positions and Radiologic Procedures.* The chapters in this workbook are presented in the same order as the 27 units in *Mosby's Radiographic Instructional Series: Anatomy, Positioning, and Procedures* multimedia and the first 27 chapters of *Merrill's Atlas of Radiographic Positions and Radiologic Procedures.* However, the material presented in this workbook can function as a useful review for any anatomy and positioning course or as a review for the certification exam.

The exercises in this revised second edition have been designed to give you a thorough review of osteology, anatomy, physiology, arthrology, and radiographic examinations.

The following features have been revised or newly added to this edition:

- Updated and standardized anatomy terminology to reflect the usage in *Merrill's Atlas* as well as the most current anatomy texts and *Nomina Anatomica*
- New questions on computed radiography (CR), including the slight positioning changes and the kVp setting changes necessary for CR
- New exercise sections on radiographic quality in Chapter 1, identifying projections of the vertebral column in Chapter 8, and review of essential mammographic projections in Chapter 24
- New chapter review self-tests for Chapters 20 through 23
- More film evaluations, offering additional opportunities to evaluate images for proper positioning
- More positioning questions to complement the workbook's strong anatomy review
- Reformatted exercises for ease of writing in answers while working through the *MRIS* multimedia tutorials

The chapters that include essential projections are divided into two sections: (1) an anatomy section and (2) a positioning section.

- The anatomy sections consist of various exercises such as labeling and identification diagrams, short-answer and multiple-choice questions, matching exercises, and crossword puzzles.
- The positioning sections include short-answer and multiple-choice questions, true-false statements, fill-in-the-blank statements, matching exercises, identification exercises, and radiographic comparisons of standard radiographic projections.
- The last exercise in each chapter, a self-test, is a collection of multiple-choice questions to review the entire chapter. All answers for exercises are found at the end of each volume.

Some of the radiographic projections included and described in *Merrill's Atlas* are for reference purposes only and are no longer routinely performed in radiologic imaging facilities. Therefore, we have chosen to focus on essential terminology, anatomy, and positioning information for the projections identified as necessary for entry-level competency as determined by a survey of radiologic technology programs in the United States and Canada. For more information on the survey, consult the Preface contained in *Merrill's Atlas.*

Some chapters of *Merrill's Atlas* (Volumes 1 and 2) have limited radiographic applications or comprise radiographic procedures only rarely performed today because of technological advances in adjunct medical imagery modalities (e.g., computed tomography, magnetic resonance imaging, and diagnostic ultrasound). Because those chapters do not include radiographic examinations deemed to be essential for entry-level competency, this workbook provides only cursory coverage for those chapters.

To use this workbook most effectively, you should complete each set of exercises after studying the appropriate anatomic and radiographic sections from *Merrill's Atlas* and the multimedia series. Answers to the exercises are provided at the end of each volume so you can check your progress.

Steven G. Hayes Sr.

Acknowledgments

My appreciation is extended to those who were instrumental in the development of this workbook. The first, of course, is my wife Sharon. The simple dedication in the front of this workbook does not adequately express my appreciation for all her support and assistance with this publication and with every goal I ever pursued. For more than 30 years she has given me more than I can ever return in kind.

The difficulties of a major writing project are, sometimes, not fully realized by an author upon initially accepting the task. Support from family members can often affect how successful an author is in completing a publication. I am fortunate to have the complete support of my family. For that reason I need to recognize my two children who allowed me to temporarily withdraw my presence from their activities. My son, Steven G. Hayes Jr., ASRT, RT(R) (ARRT), is very supportive of everything I do, especially with the development of this workbook. Because he is an experienced radiologic educator and technologist, his knowledge of radiographic positioning was very beneficial to me in obtaining some of the radiographic images I needed and with assisting in the development of the text. I value his support and advice. I also want to thank my daughter, Tonya, for her understanding when I was excusing myself from family activities so I could sustain my production schedule. To both, I apologize for depriving them of my time during the development of this workbook.

Another radiologic educator, Jackie Miller, BSRT, RT(R) (ARRT), has been a close friend and colleague of mine longer than either of us can remember. I know no one who has more common sense than Jackie. Other than my wife, he probably knows me better than does anyone else. I appreciate his assistance with obtaining some of the radiographs used in this workbook and the long-term encouragement he has given me in all my endeavors.

I also want to recognize my Mosby editors: Jeanne Rowland, Lisa Potts, and Carole Glauser. Jeanne is the acquisitions editor who first proposed this workbook project to me. I appreciate the confidence she had in me from the very onset. Lisa, an accomplished developmental editor, was very important in assisting me throughout the entire development of the first edition of this workbook. She was always available to answer every question I had and provided useful advice that made my work so much easier. Thank you, Lisa. For the preparation of this second edition, I thank Carole Glauser for coordinating the many activities that transforms a manuscript into the finished publication.

I also thank Philip W. Ballinger, MS, RT, FAERS, and Eugene Frank, MA, RT(R), FASRT, co-authors for *Merrill's Atlas of Radiographic Positions and Radiologic Procedures,* ninth edition. Philip was quick to answer my technical questions concerning Merrill's Atlas and offered significant suggestions. For the preparation of this second edition, in addition to Philip, I thank Eugene for his replies to my countless e-mail messages I sent him almost nightly for months as this revision neared its completion.

For the preparation of this second edition, in addition to the above, I sincerely appreciate the comments and suggestions from students, educators, and reviewers. Their collective input helped make this workbook a better learning aid.

I have been lucky to have the love and support of many wonderful people. Those I have just mentioned are the ones who really are responsible for this workbook.

Steven G. Hayes Sr.

Contents

Volume One

CHAPTER 1 Preliminary Steps in Radiography, 1

CHAPTER 2 Radiation Protection, 15

CHAPTER 3 General Anatomy and Radiographic Positioning Terminology, 21

CHAPTER 4 Upper Limb (Extremity), 51

CHAPTER 5 Shoulder Girdle, 95

CHAPTER 6 Lower Limb (Extremity), 113

CHAPTER 7 Pelvis and Upper Femora, 159

CHAPTER 8 Vertebral Column, 177

CHAPTER 9 Bony Thorax, 233

CHAPTER 10 Thoracic Viscera, 257

CHAPTER 11 Long Bone Measurement, 283

CHAPTER 12 Contrast Arthrography, 287

CHAPTER 13 Foreign-Body Localization and Trauma Radiography Guidelines, 291

ANSWERS TO EXERCISES

Chapter 1, 297
Chapter 2, 298
Chapter 3, 298
Chapter 4, 301
Chapter 5, 305
Chapter 6, 308
Chapter 7, 314
Chapter 8, 316
Chapter 9, 321
Chapter 10, 324
Chapter 11, 327
Chapter 12, 327
Chapter 13, 327

Volume Two

CHAPTER 14 Mouth and Salivary Glands, 1

CHAPTER 15 Anterior Part of the Neck, 9

CHAPTER 16 Digestive System: Abdomen, Liver, Spleen, and Biliary Tract, 15

CHAPTER 17 Digestive System: Alimentary Tract, 37

CHAPTER 18 Urinary System, 75

CHAPTER 19 Reproductive System, 99

CHAPTER 20 Skull, 111

CHAPTER 21 Facial Bones, 159

CHAPTER 22 Paranasal Sinuses, 181

CHAPTER 23 Temporal Bone, 195

CHAPTER 24 Mammography, 203

CHAPTER 25 Central Nervous System, 209

CHAPTER 26 Circulatory System, 217

CHAPTER 27 Sectional Anatomy for Radiographers, 237

APPENDIX Supplemental Exercises for Skull Positioning, 263

ANSWERS TO EXERCISES

Chapter 14, 271
Chapter 15, 271
Chapter 16, 272
Chapter 17, 274
Chapter 18, 278
Chapter 19, 280
Chapter 20, 281
Chapter 21, 286
Chapter 22, 288
Chapter 23, 289
Chapter 24, 289
Chapter 25, 290
Chapter 26, 291
Chapter 27, 293

ANSWERS TO APPENDIX, 295

Mouth and Salivary Glands

Review

Instructions: This exercise provides an anatomic review of the mouth and salivary glands and a cursory review of sialography. Identify structures, fill in missing words, provide a short answer, match columns, select the best choice, or choose true or false (explaining any statement you believe to be false) for each item.

1. Identify each lettered structure shown in Fig. 14-1.

   A. _____

   B. _____

   C. _____

   D. _____

   E. _____

   F. _____

   G. _____

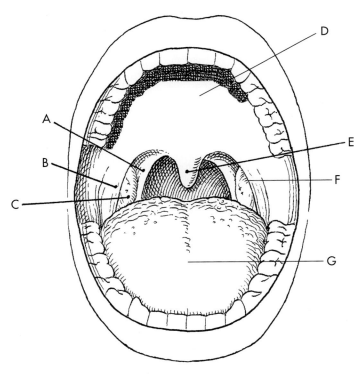

Fig. 14-1 Anterior aspect of the oral cavity.

2. Identify each lettered structure shown in Fig. 14-2.

   A. _____

   B. _____

   C. _____

   D. _____

3. Identify each lettered structure shown in Fig. 14-3.

   A. _____

   B. _____

   C. _____

   D. _____

   E. _____

   F. _____

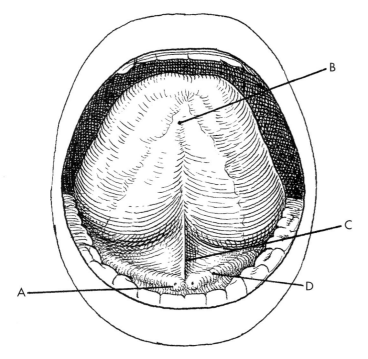

Fig. 14-2 Anterior view of the undersurface of tongue and floor of mouth.

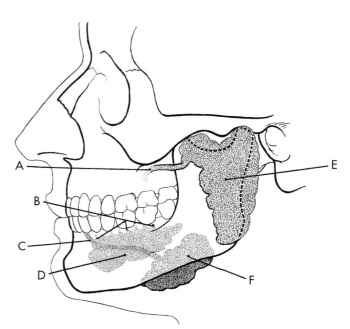

Fig. 14-3 The salivary glands from the left lateral aspect.

4. Identify each lettered structure shown in Fig. 14-4.

   A. _____

   B. _____

   C. _____

   D. _____

   E. _____

   F. _____

   G. _____

5. Identify each lettered structure shown in Fig. 14-5.

   A. _____

   B. _____

   C. _____

   D. _____

   E. _____

   F. _____

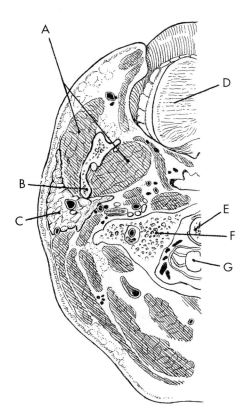

Fig. 14-4 Horizontal section of the face showing the relation of the parotid gland to the mandibular ramus. (The auricle is not shown on this illustration.)

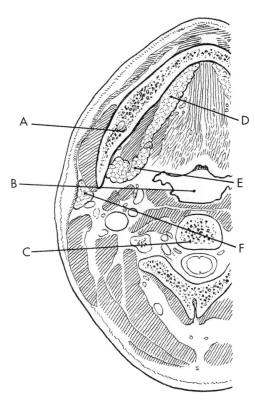

Fig. 14-5 Horizontal section of the face showing the relation of the submandibular and sublingual glands to surrounding structures. (The auricle is not shown in this illustration.)

6. What is the first division of the digestive system?

_____

7. Define *mastication.*

8. Which structures function in mastication?

_____

9. What is the purpose of saliva?

10. Name the three pairs of salivary glands.

11. Define *sialography.*

12. What type of contrast medium is used for sialography?

_____

13. Why can only one salivary gland at a time be examined by the sialographic method?

14. List two reasons that preliminary radiographs are made before the introduction of the contrast medium.

15. Name the three projections that demonstrate the salivary glands and ducts.

16. Which salivary glands are demonstrated with the axial projection (intraoral method)?
    a. Parotid and sublingual
    b. Parotid and submandibular
    c. Sublingual and submandibular

17. Which sialographic projection is the only projection that demonstrates an unobstructed image of the sublingual gland area?
    a. Lateral
    b. Tangential
    c. Axial (intraoral method)

18. Which sialographic image can be made with occlusal film?
    a. Lateral
    b. Tangential
    c. Axial (intraoral method)

19. Which sialographic projection directs the central ray along the lateral surface of the mandibular ramus?
    a. Lateral
    b. Tangential
    c. Axial (intraoral method)

20. True or False. The patient may be positioned prone or supine for the tangential projection.

21. True or False. The mandibular ramus should be parallel with the plane of the cassette for the tangential projection.

22. True or False. Parotid glands on both sides of the face should be demonstrated with the same tangential exposure.

23. Examine Fig. 14-6 and answer the questions that follow.

Fig. 14-6 Sialogram showing opacification of a gland.

a. Which projection does this image represent?

_____

b. Which salivary gland is demonstrated?

_____

c. What is the special breathing technique that can be performed by the patient to improve the radiographic demonstration of the gland with this type of projection?

24. Examine Fig. 14-7 and answer the questions that follow.

Fig. 14-7 Sialogram showing opacification of a gland.

a. Which projection does this image represent?

_____

b. Which salivary gland is demonstrated?

_____

c. To which duct does the arrow point?

_____

25. Examine Fig. 14-8 and answer the questions that follow.

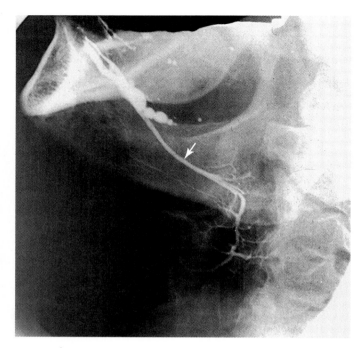

Fig. 14-8 Sialogram showing opacification of a gland.

a. Which projection does this image represent?

_____

b. Which salivary gland is demonstrated?

_____

c. To which duct does the arrow point?

_____

Self-Test: Mouth and Salivary Glands

Instructions: Answer the following questions by selecting the best choice.

1. What is the first division of the digestive system?
    a. Mouth
    b. Stomach
    c. Small intestine
    d. Salivary glands

2. Which salivary gland is the largest?
    a. Parotid
    b. Sublingual
    c. Submandibular

3. Which salivary glands are the smallest?
    a. Parotid
    b. Sublingual
    c. Submandibular

4. Which salivary glands are located along the lateral aspect of the mandibular ramus?
    a. Parotid
    b. Sublingual
    c. Submandibular

5. Which two imaging modalities have greatly reduced the frequency of sialography?
    a. Computed tomography and ultrasonography
    b. Computed tomography and magnetic resonance imaging
    c. Conventional tomography and ultrasonography
    d. Conventional tomography and magnetic resonance imaging

6. For sialography, into which structure is the contrast medium injected?
    a. Vein
    b. Artery
    c. Muscle
    d. Salivary duct

7. Which sialographic projection directs the central ray along the mandibular ramus?
    a. Lateral projection
    b. Tangential projection
    c. Verticosubmental projection
    d. Axial projection (intraoral method)

8. Which sialographic projection demonstrates a parotid gland superimposed over a mandibular ramus?
    a. Lateral projection
    b. Tangential projection
    c. Verticosubmental projection
    d. Axial projection (intraoral method)

9. Which two sialographic projections best demonstrate the parotid gland?
    a. Axial and lateral projections
    b. Axial and verticosubmental projections
    c. Tangential and lateral projections
    d. Tangential and verticosubmental projections

10. Which sialographic projection demonstrates an unobstructed view of the sublingual area?
    a. Lateral projection
    b. Tangential projection
    c. Verticosubmental projection
    d. Axial projection (intraoral method)

11. Which gland is demonstrated with tangential projections?
    a. Parotid
    b. Sublingual
    c. Submandibular

12. Which sialographic projection demonstrates parotid and submandibular glands?
    a. Lateral projection
    b. Tangential projection
    c. Axial projection (intraoral method)

13. Which salivary gland can be demonstrated with a lateral projection when the patient's head is adjusted so that the midsagittal plane is rotated approximately 15 degrees toward the cassette from true lateral and the central ray is directed to a point 1 inch (2.5 cm) above the mandibular ramus?
    a. Parotid
    b. Sublingual
    c. Submandibular

14. Which salivary gland can be demonstrated with a lateral projection when the patient's head is positioned true lateral and a perpendicular central ray is directed to the inferior margin of the mandibular angle?
    a. Parotid
    b. Sublingual
    c. Submandibular

15. For the lateral projection demonstrating the submandibular gland, what is the purpose of pressing the tongue to the floor of the mouth?
    a. To hold the intraoral film in place
    b. To displace the submandibular gland below the mandible
    c. To prevent the tongue from superimposing the submandibular gland

If your school has access to Mosby's Radiographic Instructional Series on Anatomy, Positioning, and Procedures, review Unit 14 at this time. Your instructor may request that you respond to the series' exercises on paper. This unit covers the following examinations:

Sialography
Parotid gland
Parotid and submandibular glands
Submandibular and sublingual glands

CHAPTER 15

Anterior Part of the Neck

Review

Instructions: This exercise is a review of the anatomy and radiography of the anterior part of the neck. Identify structures, fill in missing words, or provide a short answer for each item.

1. Identify each lettered structure shown in Fig. 15-1.

A. _____

B. _____

C. _____

D. _____

E. _____

F. _____

G. _____

H. _____

I. _____

J. _____

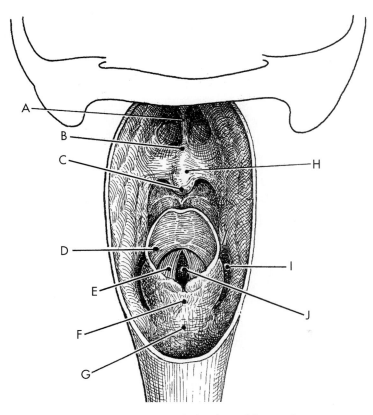

Fig. 15-1 Interior posterior view of the neck.

2. Identify each lettered structure shown in Fig. 15-2.

A. _____

B. _____

C. _____

D. _____

E. _____

F. _____

G. _____

H. _____

I. _____

J. _____

K. _____

L. _____

M. _____

Fig. 15-2 Sagittal section of the face and neck.

3. Identify each lettered structure shown in Fig. 15-3.

A. _____

B. _____

C. _____

D. _____

E. _____

F. _____

G. _____

H. _____

4. Identify each lettered structure shown in Fig. 15-4.

A. _____

B. _____

C. _____

Fig. 15-4 Anterior aspect of the larynx.

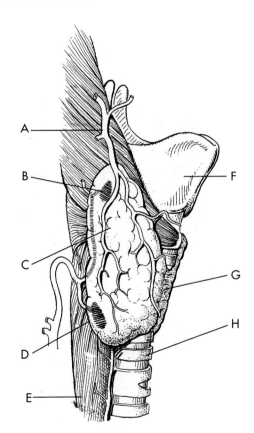

Fig. 15-3 Lateral aspect of the laryngeal area.

5. Identify each lettered structure shown in Fig. 15-5.

   A. _____

   B. _____

   C. _____

   D. _____

   E. _____

   F. _____

Fig. 15-5 Superior aspect of the larynx (open and closed true vocal folds).

6. For radiographic purposes, the neck is divided into

   _____ and

   _____ portions.

7. The upper part of the respiratory system located in the anterior part of the neck is the _____.

8. The upper part of the digestive system located in the anterior part of the neck is the _____.

9. The two major glands located in the anterior part of the neck are the _____ gland and

   _____ gland.

10. The structure of the upper neck that serves as a passage for both food and air and is common to the respiratory and digestive systems is the _____.

11. The portion of the pharynx located above the soft palate is

    the _____.

12. The portion of the pharynx located from the soft palate to

    the hyoid bone is the _____.

13. The organ of voice is the _____.

14. The structure that comprises the vocal apparatus of the larynx is the _____.

15. The projections that demonstrate the pharynx and larynx

    are _____ and

    _____.

16. During what four bodily functions are radiographs of the pharynx and larynx made?

17. Identify the body position in which the patient should be placed for each of the following examinations of the pharynx and larynx:

    a. Tomographic studies:_____

    b. AP and lateral projections: _____

18. For the AP projection, the central ray should be directed

    perpendicular to the _____

    _____.

19. Identify the x-ray tube and image receptor centering points for the lateral projection of the following structures:

    a. Nasopharynx: _____

    _____

    _____

    b. Oropharynx: _____

    _____

    _____

    c. Larynx: _____

    _____

    _____

20. Identify each lettered structure shown in Fig. 15-6.

    A. _____

    B. _____

    C. _____

    D. _____

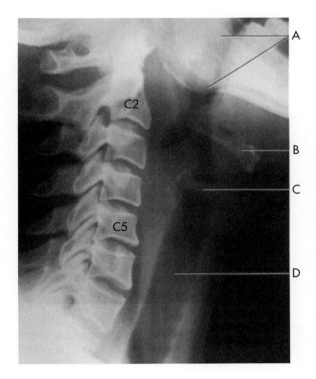

Fig. 15-6 Lateral pharynx and larynx (Valsalva maneuver).

Self-Test: Anterior Part of the Neck

Instructions: Answer the following questions by selecting the best choice.

1. What is the musculomembranous tubular structure located in front of the vertebrae and behind the nose, the mouth, and the larynx?

   a. Glottis
   b. Trachea
   c. Pharynx
   d. Esophagus

2. Which structure of the neck is approximately $1\frac{1}{2}$ inches (4 cm) in length and is situated below the root of the tongue and in front of the laryngeal pharynx?

   a. Larynx
   b. Trachea
   c. Esophagus
   d. Oropharynx

3. Which structure forms the laryngeal prominence?

   a. Epiglottis
   b. True vocal cord
   c. Cricoid cartilage
   d. Thyroid cartilage

4. Which structure prevents leakage into the larynx during swallowing?

   a. Pharynx
   b. Epiglottis
   c. Cricoid cartilage
   d. Thyroid cartilage

5. What is the most superiorly located structure of the neck?

   a. Larynx
   b. Glottis
   c. Pharynx
   d. Epiglottis

6. For the AP projection that demonstrates the pharynx and larynx, to which level of the patient should the central ray be directed?

   a. C1
   b. C7
   c. Mandibular angles
   d. Laryngeal prominence

7. For preliminary AP and lateral projections that demonstrate the pharynx and larynx, when should the exposures be made to ensure filling the throat passages with air?

   a. During expiration
   b. During inspiration
   c. After suspended expiration
   d. After suspended inspiration

8. Which body position should be used for tomographic examinations of the pharynx and larynx?

   a. Prone
   b. Supine
   c. Upright lateral
   d. Recumbent lateral

9. For the lateral projection that demonstrates the oropharynx, to which level of the patient should the central ray be directed?

   a. C7
   b. Mandibular angles
   c. Laryngeal prominence
   d. External acoustic meatuses

10. Which procedure should be performed by the patient for tomographic studies of pharyngolaryngeal structures?

    a. Quiet inspiration through the nose
    b. Phonation of a high-pitched "e-e-e"
    c. Suspended respiration after expiration
    d. Suspended respiration after inspiration

 If your school has access to Mosby's Radiographic Instructional Series on Anatomy, Positioning, and Procedures, review Unit 15 at this time. Your instructor may request that you respond to the series' exercises on paper. This unit covers the following examinations:

Soft palate, pharynx, and larynx: alternative examination methods
   Palatography
   Nasopharyngography
   Pharyngography
   Laryngopharyngography
   Tomolaryngography
   Positive-contrast laryngopharyngography
Thyroid gland
Pharynx and larynx
Soft palate, pharynx, and larynx: radiographic examination

CHAPTER 16

Digestive System: Abdomen, Liver, Spleen, and Biliary Tract

SECTION 1

Anatomy of the Abdomen, Liver, Spleen, and Biliary Tract

Exercise 1

Instructions: This exercise pertains to the abdominal contents. Identify structures for each question.

1. Identify each lettered structure shown in Fig. 16-1.

A. _____

B. _____

C. _____

D. _____

E. _____

F. _____

G. _____

H. _____

I. _____

J. _____

K. _____

L. _____

M. _____

N. _____

O. _____

P. _____

Q. _____

R. _____

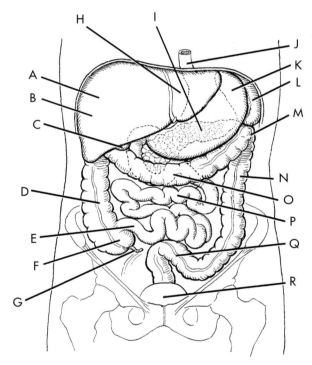

Fig. 16-1 Anterior aspect of the abdominal viscera.

2. Identify each lettered structure shown in Fig. 16-2.

A. _____

B. _____

C. _____

D. _____

E. _____

F. _____

G. _____

H. _____

I. _____

J. _____

K. _____

L. _____

M. _____

N. _____

O. _____

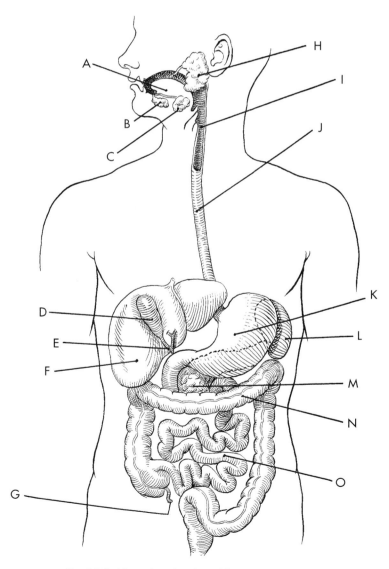

Fig. 16-2 Alimentary tract and its accessory organs.

3. Identify each lettered structure shown in Fig. 16-3.

A. _____   I. _____

B. _____   J. _____

C. _____   K. _____

D. _____   L. _____

E. _____   M. _____

F. _____   N. _____

G. _____   O. _____

H. _____

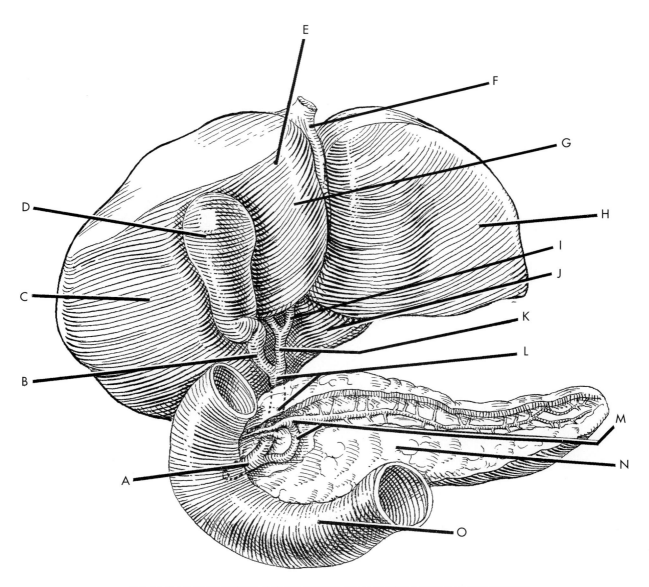

Fig. 16-3 Visceral surface (inferoposterior aspect) of the liver and gallbladder.

4. Identify each lettered structure shown in Fig. 16-4.

    A. _____

    B. _____

    C. _____

    D. _____

    E. _____

    F. _____

    G. _____

    H. _____

    I. _____

    J. _____

5. Identify each lettered structure shown in Fig. 16-5.

    A. _____

    B. _____

    C. _____

    D. _____

    E. _____

    F. _____

    G. _____

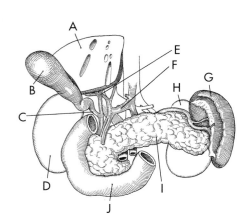

Fig. 16-4 Visceral (inferoposterior) surface of gallbladder and bile ducts.

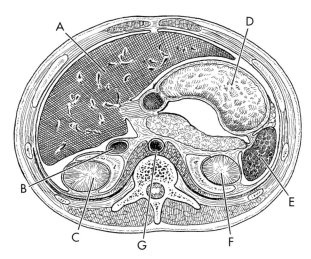

Fig. 16-5 Sectional image of the upper abdomen showing the relationship of digestive system components.

Exercise 2

Instructions: This exercise pertains to the liver, biliary system, pancreas, and spleen. Fill in missing words, provide a short answer, or choose true or false (explaining any statement you believe to be false) for each item.

1. The name of the double-walled seromembranous sac that lines the abdominal cavity is the

   _____.

2. The names of the two layers of the peritoneum are the

   _____ layer and

   _____ layer.

3. The outer layer of the peritoneum that contacts the underside of the diaphragm is called the

   _____ layer.

4. The inner layer of the peritoneum that contacts various organs is called the _____ layer.

5. The organ that occupies most of the right hypochondrium and the epigastrium regions of the abdomen is the

   _____.

6. The largest organ in the abdominal cavity is the

   _____.

7. The radiographically significant physiologic function of

   the liver is the production of _____.

8. The right and left hepatic ducts join to form the

   _____ _____

   _____.

9. The cystic duct enables bile from the liver to be stored in

   the _____.

10. The gallbladder is usually located on the inferior side of

    the right lobe of the _____.

11. The common hepatic duct unites with the cystic duct to

    form the _____

    _____ _____.

12. In 20% of subjects, before entering the duodenum, the common bile duct joins with the

    _____ _____.

13. The muscular contraction of the gallbladder is activated by

    a hormone called _____.

14. Another name for the ampulla of Vater is the

    _____ _____.

15. The gland that produces insulin is the

    _____.

16. True or False. In a hypersthenic patient, the gallbladder is situated high and well away from the midsagittal plane.

17. True or False. The gallbladder is located posterior to the liver in the retroperitoneal space.

18. True or False. The pancreas cannot be demonstrated using plain radiography.

19. True or False. The spleen is an organ of the lymphatic system.

20. True or False. The pancreas and the liver secrete specialized digestive juices into the small intestine.

SECTION 2

Positioning of the Abdomen and Gallbladder

Exercise 1: Positioning for the Abdomen

Instructions: A variety of radiographic procedures are used to demonstrate the abdomen and its contents. A patient is usually first examined with plain radiography before specialized studies using contrast media are performed. This exercise reviews the positions and projections commonly used to produce radiographs of the abdomen without the introduction of a contrast medium. Fill in missing words, provide a short answer, select answers from a list, or choose true or false (explaining any statement you believe to be false) for each item.

Items 1 through 15 pertain to *AP and PA projections.* Examine Fig. 16-6 as you answer the following items.

Fig. 16-6 AP abdomen, supine.

1. What is the commonly used acronym that refers to AP projections of the abdomen with the patient supine?

   _____

2. For the AP projection with the patient supine, to what level of the patient should the cassette be centered?

   _____

3. List the two levels of the patient to which the cassette should be centered when the patient is positioned upright, and give the reason for the difference in cassette placement.

4. List the three considerations for the use of gonadal shielding in abdominal radiography.

5. An excellent criterion for judging the quality of an abdominal radiograph is whether the outline of the

   _____ muscle is seen to be sharply defined.

6. Exposure of abdominal radiographs should be made after

   suspending _____ (inspiration or expiration).

7. Explain why the exposure should not be made for 1 or 2 seconds after respiration is suspended.

8. Which plane of the body should be centered to the midline of the cassette?

_____

9. What structure of the upper abdomen should be seen on the radiograph when the patient is upright? Explain why.

10. What two identification markers should be seen on the radiograph when the patient is upright?

11. With reference to radiation protection, what is the advantage of the PA projection over the AP projection?

12. What three projections usually comprise the three-way or acute abdomen series?

13. Why is a chest radiograph included as part of the acute abdomen series?

14. In the acute abdomen series, what radiograph should be substituted for the upright abdomen radiograph when the patient is unable to stand?

_____

15. From the list below, circle the three evaluation criteria that indicate the patient was properly positioned without rotation for a KUB radiograph.

   a. Intervertebral foramina should be open
   b. Alae or wings of the ilia should be symmetric
   c. Lumbar vertebrae pedicles should be superimposed
   d. If seen, ischial spines of the pelvis should be symmetric
   e. Spinous processes should be in the center of the lumbar vertebrae

Items 16 through 26 pertain to the *AP projection, left lateral decubitus position.* Examine Fig. 16-7 as you answer the following items.

Fig. 16-7 AP abdomen, left lateral decubitus position.

16. What is the advantage of the left lateral decubitus position compared to the supine position?

17. Why is the left lateral decubitus position preferred over the right lateral decubitus position when the patient is unable to stand?

18. Describe the position of the patient for left lateral decubitus position.

19. Why is it advisable to let the patient remain in the lateral recumbent position for several minutes before making the exposure?

20. With reference to the patient, describe the placement and centering of the cassette.

21. What breathing instructions should be given to the patient?

22. Describe how and to where the central ray should be directed.

23. Which side of the abdomen—the "up" side or the "down" side—should be demonstrated if only one side can be imaged and the patient may have free air in the abdomen?

_____

24. Which side of the abdomen—the "up" side or the "down" side—should be demonstrated if only one side can be imaged and the patient is suspected of having fluid levels within the abdominal cavity?

_____

25. What structure of the upper abdomen should be demonstrated on the radiograph?

_____

26. What identification markers should be seen on the radiograph?

Items 27 through 33 pertain to the _lateral projection_. Examine Fig. 16-8 as you anwer the following items.

Fig. 16-8 Right lateral abdomen.

27. True or False. A lateral projection of the abdomen can be performed with the patient placed in either the right lateral recumbent position or the left lateral recumbent position.

28. True or False. The exposure should be made after the patient has suspended respiration after full inspiration.

29. True or False. The midsagittal plane should be perpendicular and centered to the cassette.

30. To what level of the patient should the cassette be centered?

31. If a compression band is needed to immobilize the patient, where should it be placed?

32. Where exactly should the central ray enter the patient?

33. What two areas of the image can be closely examined to determine if the patient was rotated?

_____

Items 34 through 40 pertain to the *lateral projection, dorsal decubitus position.* Examine Fig. 16-9 as you answer the following items.

Fig. 16-9 Lateral abdomen, left dorsal decubitus position.

34. What is the name of the radiographic position that produces a lateral image of the abdomen with the patient in the supine position?

_____

35. To what level of the patient should the long axis of the cassette be centered?

_____

36. How far above the level of the iliac crests should the central ray enter the patient?

_____

37. What purpose is served by having the patient slightly flex his or her knees?

38. True or False. The exposure should be made after the patient has suspended respiration at the end of inspiration.

39. True or False. The central ray should be directed horizontally and perpendicular relative to the center of the film.

40. From the list below, circle the three evaluation criteria that indicate the patient was correctly positioned for a lateral projection while placed in the dorsal decubitus position.
    a. The wings of the ilia should be symmetric.
    b. The entire abdomen should be demonstrated.
    c. The diaphragm should be included without motion.
    d. The abdominal contents should be seen with soft tissue gray tones.
    e. The spinous processes should be seen in the center of the lumbar vertebrae.
    f. The ribs and pelvis should be equidistant to the edge of the cassette on both sides.

Exercise 2: Contrast Studies for the Gallbladder

Instructions: This exercise pertains to radiographic demonstrations of the gallbladder using a contrast medium. Fill in missing words, provide a short answer, or choose true or false (explaining any statement you believe to be false) for each item.

1. Radiographic visualization of the gallbladder after the introduction of a contrast medium is termed

   _____.

2. The most common method by which a contrast medium is introduced into a patient for cholecystography is the

   _____ method.

3. Two common abbreviations for oral cholecystography are

   ____ and ____.

4. An oral cholecystopaque is absorbed through the intestines and transported to the liver by the

   _____ vein.

5. Define the following terms.

   a. Cholelithiasis: _____

      _____

      _____

   b. Choledocholithiasis: _____

      _____

      _____

   c. Cholecystitis: _____

      _____

      _____

   d. Biliary stenosis: _____

      _____

      _____

6. The most common pathologic reason for performing oral cholecystography (OCG) is to demonstrate

   _____.

7. List six topics that should be included in written instructions given to patients preparing for OCG.

8. After a patient arrives in the radiography department for an OCG examination, why is it important to determine whether the patient experienced vomiting or diarrhea after ingesting the oral cholecystopaque tablets?

9. Why should patients be scheduled for OCG examinations in the early part of the morning?

10. What two purposes may be served by performing a general survey scout radiograph of the patient before preparation for OCG examinations?

11. If the use of a laxative is part of the preparation for an OCG examination, why should the patient be instructed *not* to use a laxative less than 24 hours before swallowing the oral cholecystopaque tablets?

12. After consuming the oral cholecystopaque tablets but before arriving in the radiography department for the scheduled OCG examination, what food or drink is the patient allowed to consume?

13. What imaging modality is often used to complement an OCG examination if gallbladder images fail to provide a diagnosis?

_____

14. True or False. Pure cholesterol gallstones appear as negative filling defects within the opacified bile.

15. True or False. Gallstones containing calcium can often be seen on plain radiography before the introduction of a contrast medium.

Items 16 through 31 pertain to the *PA projection.* Examine Fig. 16-10 as you answer the following items.

Fig. 16-10 PA gallbladder, upright position.

16. True or False. The PA projection can be performed with the patient either in the prone position or upright.

17. True or False. The left side of the patient should be centered to the midline of the table.

18. Which focal spot size—large or small—should be used for radiography of the gallbladder?

_____

19. What is the maximum exposure time that should be used for exposing the cassettes?

_____

20. What procedure should be performed to prevent pendulous breasts of female patients from superimposing the gallbladder?

21. With the patient in the prone position, why should the left cheek (rather than the right cheek) rest on a pillow?

22. What can be done to the lower limbs to relieve pressure on the toes when the patient is prone?

23. At what point during patient breathing should the exposure be made?

24. How much time should elapse after the patient suspends respiration before the exposure is made? Explain why.

25. Examine the radiographs in Figs. 16-11 and 16-12 and answer the questions that follow.

Fig. 16-11 Gallbladder radiograph.

Fig. 16-12 Gallbladder radiograph.

a. Which radiograph was exposed after the patient suspended respiration after expiration?

b. Which radiograph should be marked to indicate the specific phase of respiration when the exposure was made?

26. What procedure should be performed for a subsequent PA projection radiograph with the patient in the prone position if the first PA projection radiograph demonstrates the gallbladder superimposed with rib shadows?

27. Identify the body habitus type—sthenic, asthenic, or hypersthenic—for which each of the following central ray centering levels is used:

a. 9th costal cartilage: _____

b. 2 inches (5 cm) above the 9th costal cartilage:

c. 2 inches (5 cm) below the 9th costal cartilage:

28. Is the centering point for the patient who has been moved to the standing position from the prone position relatively higher or lower?

29. How much does the gallbladder's position shift when a prone patient is moved to the upright position?

30. When the patient is positioned in the upright position, where should gallstones that are heavier than bile be demonstrated within the gallbladder?

31. Listed below are statements pertaining to the prone and upright positions. In the space provided, write *P* if the statement pertains to the prone position or *U* if the statement pertains to the upright position.

_____ a. This position can show different layers of gallstones.

_____ b. This position best demonstrates mobility of the gallbladder.

_____ c. This position produces a foreshortened image of the gallbladder.

_____ d. This position usually projects a more vertical image of a gallbladder.

_____ e. Radiographs of this position should be marked to indicate the position of the patient.

_____ f. This position produces an irregular circular or triangular image of the gallbladder.

_____ g. This position is best for demonstrating many gallstones that are too small to be seen individually.

_____ h. This position generally requires higher localization centering than the other PA projection.

Items 32 through 42 pertain to the *PA oblique projection (LAO position)* and the *lateral projection (right lateral position)*. Examine Figs. 16-13 and 16-14 as you answer the following items.

Fig. 16-13 PA oblique gallbladder, LAO position.

Fig. 16-14 Right lateral gallbladder.

32. The PA oblique projection (LAO position) is particularly effective in separating the shadow of the gallbladder from

the _____ _____.

33. How many degrees should the patient be rotated from the prone position for the PA oblique projection (LAO position)?

_____

34. List three factors that affect the degree of rotation when positioning the patient for the PA oblique projection (LAO position).

35. Which type of patient—thin or large—requires more rotation?

_____

36. Why should the recumbent patient be positioned LAO instead of RPO (even though both positions produce similar images)?

37. Why should a radiolucent foam wedge be placed against the anterior surface of the abdomen when the recumbent patient is placed in the LAO position?

38. Why is the right lateral position preferred over the left lateral position when the lateral projection is performed?

39. The right lateral projection is sometimes used to differentiate gallstones from _____ stones.

40. The exposure should be made after the patient has suspended respiration after _____.

41. The right lateral position is useful for separating the shadows of the gallbladder and the vertebrae for patients who are exceptionally _____ (large or thin).

42. Cholecystograms should demonstrate the gallbladder and surrounding structures in _____ (long-scale or short-scale) contrast.

Items 43 through 50 pertain to the *AP projection (right lateral decubitus position)*. Examine Fig. 16-15 as you answer the following items.

Fig. 16-15 AP gallbladder, right lateral decubitus position.

43. One advantage of this position is that the gallbladder

    should gravitate towards the _____ (right or left) side.

44. With reference to adjacent gas-containing loops of the in-

    testine, the gallbladder should lie _____ (above or below) gas shadows.

45. Which contrast scale—long or short—should be used to best demonstrate the gallbladder?

    _____

46. In addition to a side marker, what other marker should be seen on the radiograph?

    _____

47. Why should the patient be elevated 2 to 3 inches (5 to 7.5 cm) on a suitable radiolucent support?
    a. To demonstrate vertebral bodies
    b. To ensure that the diaphragm is included in the image
    c. To center the gallbladder region to the image receptor

48. Which term best describes how the central ray should be directed?
    a. Angled
    b. Vertically
    c. Horizontally

49. True or False. The right lateral decubitus position is used for stratification studies of the low-placed gallbladder.

50. True or False. The left lateral decubitus position should be used if the patient is unable to stand or be positioned for the right lateral decubitus position.

Exercise 3: Identifying Gallbladder Radiographs

Instructions: Examine the images of gallbladders in Figs. 16-16 through 16-19. Based on the appearance or the location of each gallbladder relative to its surrounding structures, identify in which position the patient was most likely placed for the exposure: PA (prone), PA (upright), left anterior oblique (LAO), or right lateral decubitus.

Fig. 16-16 Gallbladder radiograph.

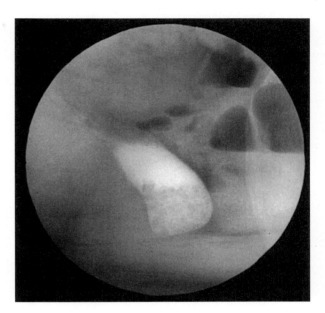

Fig. 16-17 Gallbladder radiograph.

1. Fig. 16-16: _____

2. Fig. 16-17: _____

Fig. 16-18 Gallbladder radiograph.

Fig. 16-19 Gallbladder radiograph.

3. Fig. 16-18: _____

4. Fig. 16-19: _____

Self-Test: Abdomen, Liver, Spleen, and Biliary Tract

Instructions: Answer the following questions by selecting the best choice.

1. Which organ produces bile?
   a. Liver
   b. Spleen
   c. Pancreas
   d. Gallbladder

2. Which body function is performed by the pancreas?
   a. Filtration of blood
   b. Production of bile
   c. Production of lymphocytes
   d. Production of digestive juices

3. Which organ stores and concentrates bile?
   a. Liver
   b. Spleen
   c. Pancreas
   d. Gallbladder

4. Which substance activates the muscular contraction of the gallbladder?
   a. Bile
   b. Cholecystokinin
   c. Pancreatic juices
   d. Cholecystolithiasis

5. The spleen is part of which body system?
   a. Urinary
   b. Digestive
   c. Endocrine
   d. Lymphatic

6. In which organ are clusters of islet cells found?
   a. Liver
   b. Spleen
   c. Pancreas
   d. Gallbladder

7. How many major lobes does the liver have?
   a. One
   b. Two
   c. Three
   d. Four

8. Which structure forms the mesentery and omenta folds?
   a. Liver
   b. Pancreas
   c. Gallbladder
   d. Peritoneum

9. Which organ's blood is supplied by the portal vein?
   a. Liver
   b. Spleen
   c. Pancreas
   d. Gallbladder

10. Which duct is formed by the merging of the right and left hepatic ducts?
    a. Cystic
    b. Pancreatic
    c. Common bile
    d. Common hepatic

11. Which duct is formed by the union of the cystic duct with the common hepatic duct?
    a. Pancreatic
    b. Left hepatic
    c. Right hepatic
    d. Common bile

12. Where do the pancreatic and common bile ducts terminate?
    a. Ileum
    b. Duodenum
    c. Gallbladder
    d. Large intestine

13. Which duct connects the gallbladder to the common hepatic duct?
    a. Cystic
    b. Pancreatic
    c. Right hepatic
    d. Common bile

14. Which three projections usually comprise the acute abdomen series for ambulatory patients?
    a. Supine KUB, AP upright abdomen, and PA chest
    b. Supine KUB, right lateral decubitus abdomen, and PA chest
    c. Left lateral decubitus abdomen, dorsal decubitus abdomen, and PA chest
    d. Right lateral decubitus abdomen, left lateral decubitus abdomen, and dorsal decubitus abdomen

15. To which level of the patient should the cassette be centered for the KUB?
    a. T10 vertebral body
    b. L3 vertebral body
    c. 2 inches (5 cm) above the iliac crests
    d. Iliac crests

16. For the AP upright abdomen radiograph of an adult of average size, why should the cassette be slightly raised above the centering level used for the supine KUB radiograph?
    a. To include the bladder
    b. To include the diaphragm
    c. To visualize gallstones
    d. To visualize kidney stones

17. For the KUB radiograph, when should respiration be suspended, and what effect will that have on the patient?
    a. On full expiration; elevate the diaphragm
    b. On full expiration; depress the diaphragm
    c. On full inspiration; elevate the diaphragm
    d. On full inspiration; depress the diaphragm

18. Why is it desirable to include the diaphragm in the upright abdomen radiograph?
    a. To demonstrate free air in the abdomen
    b. To demonstrate fluid levels in the thorax
    c. To demonstrate fluid levels in the abdomen
    d. To demonstrate calculi in the gallbladder and kidneys

19. Which of the following guidelines is not necessary to follow when deciding whether to use gonadal shielding for the KUB radiograph?
    a. The patient has reasonable reproductive potential.
    b. The gonads lie within 2 inches (5 cm) of the primary beam.
    c. The purpose for performing the examination is not compromised.
    d. The permission to use gonadal shielding is granted by the patient.

20. Which projection should be used to demonstrate free air within the abdominal cavity when the patient is unable to stand for an upright abdomen radiograph?
    a. AP projection with the patient supine
    b. Lateral projection, dorsal decubitus position
    c. AP projection, left lateral decubitus position
    d. AP projection, right lateral decubitus position

21. Which projection does *not* demonstrate free air levels within the abdomen?
    a. AP projection with the patient supine
    b. AP projection with the patient upright
    c. Lateral projection, dorsal decubitus position
    d. AP projection, left lateral decubitus position

22. What is the major advantage of the PA projection of the abdomen over the AP projection of the abdomen?
    a. The PA projection reduces the OID of the kidneys.
    b. The PA projection reduces the exposure dose to the gonads.
    c. The PA projection magnifies gallstones for better visualization.
    d. The PA projection demonstrates the pubic rami below the urinary bladder.

23. Which radiographic position of the abdomen requires that the patient be placed in the lateral recumbent position on his or her left side and that the central ray be directed along the midsagittal plane, entering the anterior surface of the patient's abdomen at the level of the iliac crests?
    a. Dorsal decubitus
    b. Ventral decubitus
    c. Left lateral decubitus
    d. Right lateral decubitus

24. Which radiographic position of the abdomen requires that the patient be supine and that the central ray be directed to a lateral side of the patient, entering slightly anterior to the midcoronal plane?
    a. Dorsal decubitus
    b. Ventral decubitus
    c. Left lateral decubitus
    d. Right lateral decubitus

25. Which radiographic position of the abdomen requires that the patient be placed in the lateral recumbent position on his or her left side, that the cassette be placed under the patient and centered to the abdomen at the level of the iliac crests, and that the central ray be directed to enter the right side of the patient slightly anterior to the midcoronal plane?
    a. Left lateral
    b. Right lateral
    c. Left lateral decubitus
    d. Right lateral decubitus

26. The lateral projection with the patient placed in the dorsal decubitus position, the left lateral projection, and the left lateral decubitus position of the abdomen all require which of the following?
    a. The central ray should enter the left side of the patient.
    b. The patient should suspend respiration after expiration.
    c. The patient should suspend respiration after inspiration.
    d. The central ray should enter the anterior side of the abdomen.

27. For the lateral projection with the patient placed in the dorsal decubitus position, where should the central ray enter the patient?

    a. 2 inches (5 cm) anterior to the midcoronal plane at the level of the iliac crests
    b. 2 inches (5 cm) anterior to the midcoronal plane and 2 inches above the level of the iliac crests
    c. 2 inches (5 cm) posterior to the midcoronal plane at the level of the iliac crests
    d. 2 inches (5 cm) posterior to the midcoronal plane and 2 inches above the level of the iliac crests

28. For the lateral projection with the patient placed in the dorsal decubitus position, which procedure should be performed to ensure that the entire abdomen is included on the radiograph?

    a. Use support cushions to elevate the patient.
    b. Center the cassette to the level of the xiphoid process.
    c. Center the cassette to the anterior surface of the abdomen.
    d. Direct the central ray to a point 2 inches (5 cm) below the iliac crests.

29. Which structures should be examined to see whether the patient was rotated for a lateral projection of the abdomen?

    a. Pelvis and lumbar vertebrae
    b. Pelvis and thoracic vertebrae
    c. Diaphragm and lumbar vertebrae
    d. Diaphragm and thoracic vertebrae

30. Which imaging procedure should be part of the OCG examination?

    a. Use long exposure times and long-scale contrast
    b. Use long exposure times and short-scale contrast
    c. Use short exposure times and long-scale contrast
    d. Use short exposure times and short-scale contrast

31. For oral cholecystography procedures, when should respiration be suspended, and what effect will this have on the position of the gallbladder?

    a. On full inspiration; depress the gallbladder
    b. On full inspiration; elevate the gallbladder
    c. On full expiration; depress the gallbladder
    d. On full expiration; elevate the gallbladder

32. Which procedure should be performed when the patient is rotated from a prone position to the LAO position for an OCG examination?

    a. Make the exposure after full inspiration.
    b. Center the cassette to the left side of the patient.
    c. Center the cassette to the level of the diaphragm.
    d. Place a radiolucent foam wedge under the abdomen.

33. For an OCG examination of a patient of average build, where should the cassette be centered?

    a. At the level of the 9th rib on the left side
    b. At the level of the 9th rib on the right side
    c. At the level of the 12th rib on the left side
    d. At the level of the 12th rib on the right side

34. Compared with cassette placement for a patient of average build, how should the cassette be moved for an OCG examination of a hypersthenic patient?

    a. Lower
    b. Higher
    c. To the left of the vertebral column
    d. More to the lateral side of the right side of the abdomen

35. Which procedure should be performed for a subsequent PA projection radiograph when the initial PA projection radiograph demonstrates the shadow of the gallbladder superimposed by ribs?

    a. Make the exposure after full inspiration.
    b. Use radiolucent cushions to elevate the patient.
    c. Direct the central ray caudally 10 to 15 degrees.
    d. Place the patient in the Trendelenburg position.

36. Which procedure most effectively separates the shadows of the gallbladder and vertebrae?

    a. Make the exposure after full inspiration.
    b. Rotate the patient into an oblique position.
    c. Place the patient in the Trendelenburg position.
    d. Position the patient for a dorsal decubitus projection.

37. Which projection best demonstrates the stratification of gallstones?

    a. AP projection with the patient supine
    b. PA projection with the patient prone
    c. AP projection, right lateral decubitus position
    d. PA oblique projection (RAO position) with the patient recumbent

38. Which procedure best demonstrates a gallbladder that is situated in the iliac fossa?

    a. Place the patient in the prone position.
    b. Place the patient in the supine position.
    c. Place the patient in the upright position.
    d. Make the exposure after full inspiration.

39. Why should patients be scheduled for OCG examinations in the early morning?

    a. Prolonged fasting causes the formation of gas.
    b. Scheduling conflicts with fluoroscopy are prevented.
    c. Continual production of bile dilutes the contrast medium.
    d. A gallbladder can only store contrast medium for 8 hours.

40. Which projection places the gallbladder closest to the cassette?
    a. PA projection
    b. AP projection
    c. PA oblique projection (LAO position) with the patient upright
    d. AP oblique projection (LPO position) with the patient recumbent

41. Which procedure should not be performed as part of patient preparation for the OCG examination?
    a. Administer a cleansing enema to prepare the intestinal tract.
    b. Instruct the patient to consume only water after swallowing oral contrast medium.
    c. Instruct the patient to take laxatives within 24 hours before swallowing oral contrast medium.
    d. Give the patient a fat-free evening meal to consume shortly before swallowing oral contrast medium.

42. Which diagnostic modality is most often used when an OCG examination does not adequately demonstrate a gallbladder?
    a. Sonography
    b. Nuclear medicine
    c. Computed tomography
    d. Magnetic resonance imaging

43. Which projection produces a foreshortened image of the gallbladder?
    a. Right lateral projection
    b. PA projection with the patient prone
    c. PA projection with the patient upright
    d. PA oblique projection (LAO position) with the patient upright

44. Which of the following projections does *not* increase the separation of the gallbladder shadow from the vertebrae?
    a. PA projection
    b. AP projection, right lateral decubitus position
    c. PA oblique projection (LAO position) with the patient upright
    d PA oblique projection (LAO position) with the patient recumbent

45. Which procedure should be performed for the left PA oblique projection that is part of an OCG examination?
    a. Make the exposure after full inspiration.
    b. Rotate thin patients more than large patients.
    c. Rotate large patients more than thin patients.
    d. Center the cassette to the left upper quadrant.

46. Which procedure should be performed when using the right lateral decubitus position that is part of an OCG examination?
    a. Place the patient on a radiolucent cushion.
    b. Center the cassette to the level of the iliac crests.
    c. Use a marker to indicate that the right side of the patient is the "up" side.
    d. Place the patient in the lateral recumbent position with the left side down.

47. What is an advantage to using the right lateral decubitus position for demonstration of the gallbladder?
    a. This position enables the gallbladder to be separated from the liver.
    b. This position enables the stomach to provide a homogeneous background density.
    c. This position enables the gallbladder to gravitate toward the dependent left side of the abdomen.
    d. This position enables the gallbladder to gravitate toward the dependent right side of the abdomen.

48. Which two projections best visualize the stratification of gallstones?
    a. AP supine KUB and prone PA projections
    b. AP supine KUB and upright PA projections
    c. AP, right lateral decubitus position, and prone PA projections
    d. AP, right lateral decubitus position, and upright PA projections

49. Which projection is generally not used as part of the OCG examination?
    a. PA projection
    b. PA oblique projection (LAO position)
    c. AP projection, right lateral decubitus position
    d. Lateral projection, dorsal decubitus position

50. Which projection of the gallbladder can be performed only with a horizontally directed central ray?
    a. PA projection
    b. Right lateral projection
    c. PA oblique projection (LAO position)
    d. AP projection, right lateral decubitus position

If your school has access to Mosby's Radiographic Instructional Series on Anatomy, Positioning, and Procedures, review Unit 16 at this time. Your instructor may request that you respond to the series' exercises on paper. This unit covers the following essential projections:

Abdomen
   AP projection
   PA projection, upright position
   AP projection, left lateral decubitus position
   Lateral projection, right or left
   Lateral projection, right or left dorsal decubitus position
Biliary tract and gallbladder
   PA projection
   PA oblique projection, LAO position
   Lateral projection, right only
   AP projection, right lateral decubitus position

CHAPTER 17

Digestive System: Alimentary Canal

SECTION 1

Anatomy of the Alimentary Canal

Exercise 1

Instructions: This exercise pertains to the digestive system. Identify structures for each question.

1. Identify each lettered structure shown in Fig. 17-1.

A. _____

B. _____

C. _____

D. _____

E. _____

F. _____

G. _____

H. _____

I. _____

J. _____

K. _____

L. _____

M. _____

N. _____

O. _____

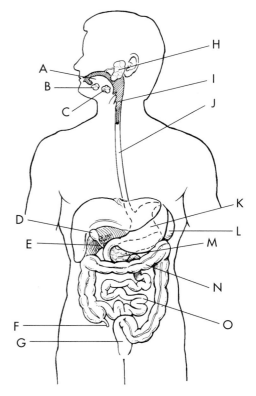

Fig. 17-1 The alimentary canal and its accessory organs.

2. Identify each lettered structure shown in Fig. 17-2.

A. _____

B. _____

C. _____

D. _____

E. _____

F. _____

G. _____

H. _____

I. _____

J. _____

K. _____

L. _____

3. Identify each lettered structure shown in Fig. 17-3.

A. _____

B. _____

C. _____

D. _____

E. _____

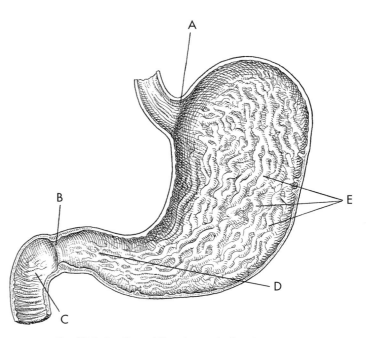

Fig. 17-3 Section of the stomach showing rugae.

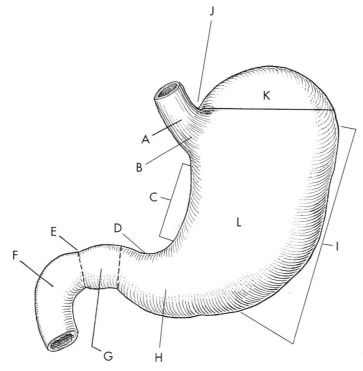

Fig. 17-2 Anterior surface of the stomach.

4. Identify each lettered structure shown in Fig. 17-4.

A. _____

B. _____

C. _____

D. _____

E. _____

F. _____

G. _____

H. _____

I. _____

J. _____

K. _____

5. Identify each lettered structure shown in Fig. 17-5.

A. _____

B. _____

C. _____

D. _____

E. _____

F. _____

G. _____

H. _____

I. _____

J. _____

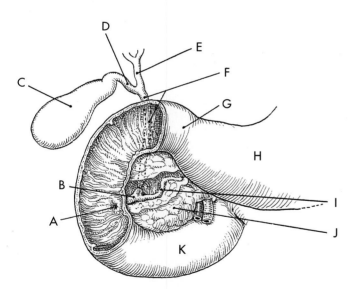

Fig. 17-4 The duodenal loop in relation to the biliary and pancreatic ducts.

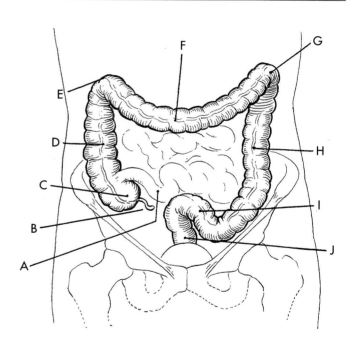

Fig. 17-5 Anterior aspect of the large bowel.

6. Identify each lettered structure shown in Fig. 17-6.

A. _____   C. _____

B. _____   D. _____

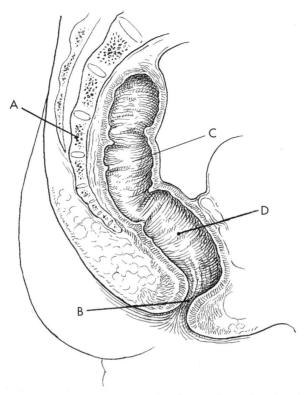

Fig. 17-6 Sagittal section showing the anal canal and rectum.

Exercise 2

Instructions: Use the following clues to complete the cross-word puzzle below. All answers refer to the alimentary canal.

ACROSS

1. Stores bile
5. Gastric folds
8. Attached to cecum
10. Terminates alimentary canal
11. Widest part of alimentary canal
15. Contraction waves
18. Proximal part of small bowel
19. Left colic flexure

22. Between cecum and right colic flexure
23. Average body build
24. Precedes anal canal

DOWN

2. Digestive juice
3. Musculomembranous tube
4. Upper part of stomach
6. Lower than sthenic

7. Proximal part of large intestine
9. Precedes esophagus
12. Large body build
13. Middle part of small bowel
14. Very slender body build
16. Intestinal bend
17. Between left colic flexure and sigmoid
20. Produces bile
21. Distal part of small bowel

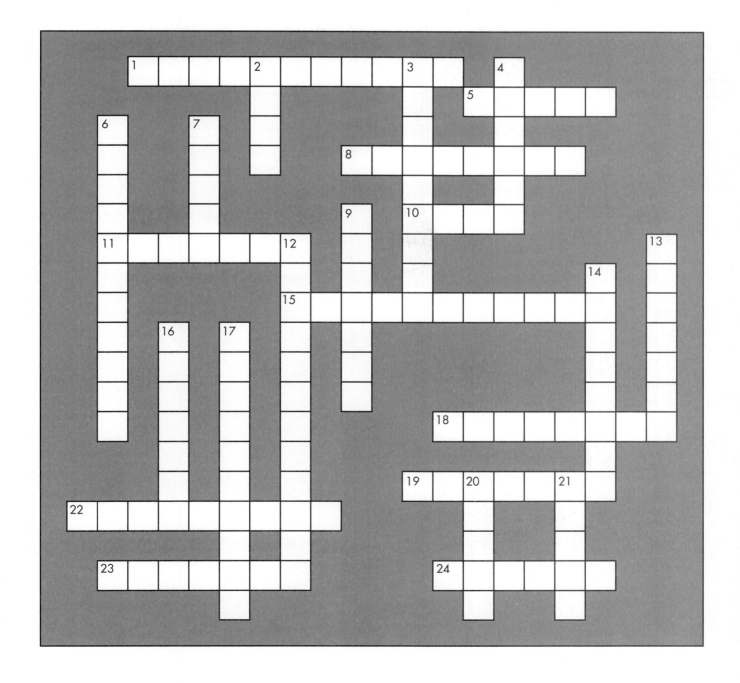

Exercise 3

Instructions: Match the structures or portions of organs found in the alimentary canal from the list in Column A with the major organs to which they most closely relate as listed in Column B.

Column A

_____ 1. Bulb

_____ 2. Body

_____ 3. Rugae

_____ 4. Ileum

_____ 5. Cecum

_____ 6. Rectum

_____ 7. Fundus

_____ 8. Pylorus

_____ 9. Sigmoid

_____ 10. Jejunum

_____ 11. Duodenum

_____ 12. Transverse

_____ 13. Ascending

_____ 14. Descending

_____ 15. Lesser curvature

_____ 16. Greater curvature

_____ 17. Ampulla of Vater

_____ 18. Cardiac sphincter

_____ 19. Left colic flexure

_____ 20. Right colic flexure

Column B

a. Stomach

b. Small intestine

c. Large intestine

Exercise 4

Instructions: This exercise pertains to the alimentary canal and its related organs. Fill in missing words or provide a short answer for each question.

1. The musculomembranous passage that extends from the pharynx to the stomach is the _____.

2. The expanded part of the distal end of the esophagus is the _____ _____.

3. The opening into the stomach through which food and liquids pass is the _____ _____.

4. The organ in which gastric digestion begins is the _____.

5. The gastric folds of the stomach are the _____.

6. The border of the stomach with the lesser curvature is the _____ border.

7. The lesser curvature extends from the esophagogastric junction to the _____.

8. The left and inferior borders of the stomach are the _____ _____.

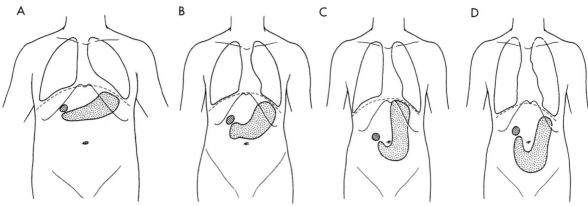

Fig. 17-7 The four types of body habitus.

9. Figure 17-7 shows four diagrams, each representing a different body habitus. Indicate in the blanks provided which of the following body habitus type each diagram represents: sthenic, asthenic, hyposthenic, or hypersthenic.

   a. Diagram A: _____

   b. Diagram B: _____

   c. Diagram C: _____

   d. Diagram D: _____

10. Name the four parts of the stomach.

11. The part of the stomach immediately surrounding the esophageal opening is the _____.

12. The most superior part of the stomach is the

    _____.

13. The most inferior part of the stomach is the

    _____ portion.

14. The opening between the stomach and the small intestine

    is the _____

    _____.

15. The three parts of the small intestine are the

    _____, _____,

    and _____.

16. The proximal part of the small intestine is the

    _____.

17. The radiographically significant first segment of the proximal part of the small intestine is the

    _____ _____.

18. The small intestine terminates at the

    _____ _____.

19. The common bile and the pancreatic ducts empty into the

    _____.

20. The middle part of the small intestine is the

    _____.

21. The distal part of the small intestine is the

    _____.

22. The shortest part the small intestine is the

    _____; the longest part is the

    _____.

23. The longer of the two intestines is the

_____ intestine.

24. The passage from the small intestine to the large intestine

is the _____

_____.

25. The proximal part of the large intestine is the

_____.

26. The veriform appendix attaches to the large intestine at the

_____.

27. Located between the ascending colon and the transverse

colon is the _____

_____ flexure.

28. The part of the colon that extends from the cecum to the

right colic flexure is the _____ colon.

29. The part of the colon that extends between the two flexures

is the _____ colon.

30. Located between the transverse colon and the descending

colon is the _____

_____ flexure.

31. The part of the colon that extends inferiorly from the left

colic flexure is the _____ colon.

32. The sigmoid colon is located between the two parts of the

large intestine known as the _____

_____ and the

_____.

33. The sigmoid colon terminates in the

_____.

34. The part of the large intestine that extends between the rec-

tum and the anus is the _____

_____.

35. The external opening at the terminal end of the anal canal

is the _____.

SECTION 2

Positioning of the Alimentary Canal

Exercise 1: Positioning for the Esophagus

Instructions: The esophagus can be radiographically examined after a contrast medium has been introduced. This exercise pertains to procedures used to obtain the required radiographs of the esophagus. Fill in missing words, provide a short answer, or choose true or false (explaining any statement you believe to be false) for each item.

1. List the projections that comprise the typical esophageal study.

2. What two types of contrast media are used for double-contrast esophageal studies?

3. Why is the left PA oblique projection (left anterior oblique [LAO] position) not included in the typical esophageal study?

4. When demonstrating the entire esophagus, to what level of the patient should the cassette be centered?

5. What two oblique positions can be used to demonstrate the entire esophagus effectively?

6. Why is the recumbent right anterior oblique (RAO) position preferred over the upright position?

7. For AP or PA projections, how is it determined that the selection of exposure factors was acceptable?

8. In relation to the surrounding structures, where should the esophagus appear in images with the patient in the RAO position?

9. In radiographs of a contrast-filled esophagus with the patient in the RAO position, how does the esophagus appear in relation to the surrounding structures when rotation of the patient was *insufficient?*

10. In the lateral projection radiograph, what structures are used to determine whether the patient was rotated? How should these structures appear?

11. For radiographs with the patient in the RAO position, the patient should be rotated approximately ____ to ____ degrees.

12. The esophagus should be clearly seen from the lower neck to the _____

_____.

13. True or False. Single-contrast and double-contrast studies can be used to demonstrate the esophagus.

14. True or False. A barium sulfate mixture is the preferred contrast medium for esophagrams.

15. True or False. The most important requirement for the contrast medium is that the weight per volume should be rated greater than 50%.

Exercise 2: The Gastrointestinal Series

Instructions: One of the more commonly performed studies employing contrast media is the gastrointestinal (GI) series. This exercise pertains to gastrointestinal studies. Identify structures, fill in missing words, provide a short answer, select from a list, or choose true or false (explaining any statement you believe to be false) for each item.

Items 1 through 20 pertain to upper gastrointestinal examination procedures.

1. What two acronyms refer to the routine upper gastrointestinal series?

_____

2. As part of patient preparation, why should the patient maintain a soft, low-residue diet for two days?

3. How can the UGI study be affected if the patient smokes cigarettes shortly before the examination?

4. What type of radiopaque contrast medium usually is used in routine UGI studies?

5. List the two general GI examination procedures routinely used to examine the stomach.

6. What is the range of weight per volume concentration for the barium sulfate suspension usually used for single-contrast examinations?

_____

7. What are the two types of contrast media used in double-contrast procedures?

8. List two advantages of performing the double-contrast examination.

9. True or False. Both the single-contrast and double-contrast procedures should begin with the patient in the lateral recumbent position.

10. True or False. The barium sulfate suspension used for double-contrast examinations should have a higher weight per volume ratio than the barium sulfate suspension used for single-contrast examinations.

11. True or False. After the patient consumes the barium sulfate suspension for a double-contrast examination, all radiographs should be performed with the patient in the upright position.

12. Why should patients undergoing double-contrast examinations turn from side-to-side or roll over a few times during the procedure?

13. What is the purpose of using glucagon during the double-contrast examination?

14. During double-contrast examinations, what instructions should be given to the patient after the patient swallows the carbon dioxide crystals or tablets to ensure a double-contrast effect?

15. What is a biphasic GI examination?

16. Which method of examination—the single-contrast or double-contrast—is performed first as part of a biphasic examination?

_____

17. What are the two methods of performing hypotonic duodenography?

18. True or False. Hypotonic duodenography originally required that the contrast medium be introduced directly through a tube placed into the duodenum.

19. True or False. The tubeless hypotonic duodenography examination is performed after the duodenum has been temporarily paralyzed by a drug.

20. True or False. Hypotonic duodenography has largely been replaced by other imaging modalities such as sonography and computed tomography.

Items 21 through 31 pertain to the *PA projection*. Examine Fig. 17-8 as you answer the following items.

Fig. 17-8 PA stomach and duodenum.

21. True or False. Routine radiographs of the stomach and duodenum should be made with the patient in the upright position.

22. True or False. The PA projection with the patient in the prone position demonstrates the contour of the barium-filled stomach and duodenal bulb.

23. True or False. The PA projection with the patient in the upright position shows the size, shape, and relative position of the barium-filled stomach.

24. True or False. A compression band may be placed across the patient's abdomen to immobilize the patient and reduce involuntary movement of the viscera.

25. How should the prone position of the patient be adjusted to prevent the full weight of the abdomen from causing the stomach and duodenum to press against the vertebral column?

26. To what point on the patient should a 24 × 30 cm (10 × 12 in) cassette be centered?

27. To what point on the patient should a 35 × 43 cm (14 × 17 in) cassette be centered?

28. How should the centering of the cassette be adjusted if the patient is repositioned from the prone position to the upright position?

29. The greatest visceral movement between the prone position and the upright position occurs in the

    _____ body habitus.

30. The central ray should be directed perpendicularly to enter

    the patient at the level of _____.

31. The exposure should be made after the patient has suspended breathing at the end of

    _____.

Items 32 through 37 pertain to the *PA oblique projection (RAO position)*. Examine Fig. 17-9 as you answer the following items.

Fig. 17-9 PA oblique stomach and duodenum, RAO position.

32. Describe how the patient should be adjusted from the prone position to the RAO position.

33. Where should the central ray enter the patient?

34. How many degrees should the patient be rotated from the prone position?
    a. 10 to 15
    b. 20 to 35
    c. 40 to 70

35. Which type of body habitus requires the most rotation?
    a. Sthenic
    b. Hyposthenic
    c. Hypersthenic

36. True or False. For the average patient, the PA oblique projection (RAO position) produces the best image of the pyloric canal and the duodenal bulb filled with barium.

37. True or False. The PA oblique projection (RAO position) radiograph should be exposed when the patient has suspended respiration after full inspiration.

Items 38 through 44 pertain to the *left AP oblique projection (left posterior oblique [LPO] position).* Examine Fig. 17-10 as you answer the following items.

Fig. 17-10 AP oblique stomach and duodenum, LPO position.

38. The left AP oblique projection (LPO position) is best performed if the patient is adjusted from the

    _____ (supine or prone) position.

39. The _____ (right or left) side of the patient should be elevated away from the table.

40. Most patients should be rotated _____ degrees for the left AP oblique projection (LPO position).

41. Where should the central ray enter the patient?

42. True or False. The left AP oblique projection (LPO position) demonstrates the fundic portion of the stomach filled with barium.

43. True or False. The left AP oblique projection (LPO position) demonstrates the pyloric canal and duodenal bulb filled with barium.

44. Identify each lettered structure shown in Fig. 17-11.

    A. _____

    B. _____

    C. _____

    D. _____

    E. _____

Fig. 17-11 AP stomach and duodenum, LPO position.

Items 45 through 50 pertain to the *right lateral projection.* Examine Fig. 17-12 as you answer the following items.

Fig. 17-12 Right lateral stomach and duodenum.

45. Which radiographic body position should be used to best demonstrate the duodenal loop and the duodenojejunal junction filled with contrast medium?

    a. Upright left lateral position
    b. Recumbent right lateral position
    c. Upright RAO position
    d. Recumbent LPO position

46. At which vertebral level should the central ray enter the patient if the patient is in the recumbent position?

    a. T10 to T11
    b. L1 to L2
    c. L5 to S1

47. At which vertebral level should the central ray enter the patient if the patient is moved from the recumbent position to the upright lateral position?

    a. T12
    b. L1
    c. L3
    d. L5

48. When examining right lateral projection radiographs, which osteologic structures should be examined to determine whether the patient was rotated?

    a. Ribs
    b. Vertebrae
    c. Pelvic bones

49. Examine Fig. 17-13 and indicate whether the following gastric structures are mostly barium-filled or mostly gas-filled:

    a. Stomach fundus: _____

    b. Duodenal bulb:_____

    c. Duodenum: _____

50. Identify each lettered structure shown in Fig. 17-13.

    A. _____

    B. _____

    C. _____

    D. _____

    E. _____

Fig. 17-13 Right lateral stomach.

Items 51 through 55 pertain to the *AP projection.* Examine Fig. 17-14 as you answer the following items.

Fig. 17-14 AP stomach and duodenum.

51. Describe the centering of the cassette for each of the following sizes.

   a. 30 × 35 cm (11 × 14 in):

   b. 35 × 43 cm (14 × 17 in):

52. Which body position should be used?

   a. Prone
   b. Supine
   c. Upright

53. Which procedure should be performed to help demonstrate a diaphragmatic herniation (hiatal hernia)?

   a. Place the patient in the upright position.
   b. Tilt the table to Fowler's angulation.
   c. Place the patient in the right lateral recumbent position.
   d. Tilt the table to the Trendelenburg angulation.

54. How should each of the following structures be demonstrated—barium-filled or gas-filled (double contrast)?

   a. Body_____

   b. Fundus: _____

   c. Pylorus_____

   d. Duodenal bulb _____

55. Identify each lettered structure shown in Fig. 17-15.

   A. _____

   B. _____

   C. _____

   D. _____

Fig. 17-15 AP stomach and duodenum.

Exercise 3: Small Intestine Examination

Instructions: The small intestine can be radiographically examined by more than one method, often after the stomach is examined. This exercise pertains to the study of the small intestine, often referred to as the small bowel series. Provide a short answer or select the answer from a list for each item.

1. List the three methods by which a barium sulfate mixture can be administered for a small bowel series.

2. Which small bowel series method is most commonly used?
   a. Oral
   b. Enteroclysis
   c. Complete reflux

3. Which small bowel series method often requires the administration of glucagon or diazepam (Valium) to relax the intestine and reduce patient discomfort during the initial filling of the small intestine?
   a. Oral
   b. Enteroclysis
   c. Complete reflux

4. Which small bowel series method injects contrast medium through an intestinal tube?
   a. Oral
   b. Enteroclysis
   c. Complete reflux

5. How should the patient be positioned when the small intestine is to be filled by the complete reflux method?
   a. Prone
   b. Supine
   c. Lateral recumbent

6. Where in the small intestine should the tube be inserted for the enteroclysis method of performing a small bowel series?
   a. Ileum
   b. Jejunum
   c. Duodenum

7. Select the four instructions from the list below that are usually given to patients preparing for the oral method of performing a small bowel series.
   a. A cleansing enema
   b. No breakfast on the morning of the examination
   c. No evening meal the night before the examination
   d. Swallow laxatives the morning of the examination
   e. Drinking 3 to 4 glasses of water the morning of the examination
   f. Nothing by mouth after the evening meal the night before the examination
   g. A restricted diet (soft, low-residue foods) for up to two days before the examination

8. Which method of performing a small bowel series does *not* use a cleansing enema as part of patient preparation?
   a. Oral
   b. Complete reflux
   c. Enteroclysis (intubation)

9. How should the patient be placed for timed radiographs when compression of the abdominal contents is desired?
   a. Prone
   b. Supine
   c. Lateral recumbent

10. Approximately how long after the patient swallows the barium sulfate mixture should the first radiograph be made?
    a. 5 minutes
    b. 15 minutes
    c. 30 minutes

11. Approximately how long after the exposure of the first radiograph should subsequent radiographs be exposed?
    a. 5 to 10 minutes
    b. 15 to 30 minutes
    c. 35 to 45 minutes

12. Why is a time marker displayed on each radiograph taken during a small bowel series?

13. How might the oral method of small bowel examination be enhanced by giving the patient a cup of cold water during the administration of the contrast medium?

14. The visualization of which structure usually indicates adequate demonstration of the entire small intestine?

    a. Jejunum
    b. Duodenum
    c. Ileocecal valve

15. For the AP projection demonstrating the small intestine, which plane of the body should be centered to the grid?

    a. Horizontal
    b. Midsagittal
    c. Midcoronal

16. For the AP projection demonstrating the small intestine of a sthenic patient within 30 minutes after the administration of contrast, to which level of the patient should the cassette be centered?

    a. T12
    b. L2
    c. L5

17. For delayed AP projections demonstrating the small intestine of a sthenic patient, to which level of the patient should the cassette be centered?

    a. T12
    b. L2
    c. Iliac crests

18. For the AP projection, when should the exposure be made?

    a. At the end of expiration
    b. At the end of inspiration

19. How should the central ray be directed?

    a. Perpendicularly
    b. Angled caudally
    c. Angled cephalically

20. From the list below, circle the seven evaluation criteria that indicate small bowel series radiographs were properly performed.

    a. The patient should not be rotated.
    b. A time marker should be included
    c. No ribs should be seen below the diaphragm.
    d. The stomach should be included on the initial radiographs.
    e. The exposure factors should demonstrate the anatomy.
    f. The entire small intestine should be included on each radiograph.
    g. The entire alimentary canal should be included on each radiograph.
    h. The vertebral column should be in the middle of the radiograph.
    i. The examination is usually completed when barium is visualized in the cecum.
    j. The post-evacuation film is accomplished after the administration of a cleansing enema.
    k. The examination is usually completed when barium is visualized in the jejunum.

Exercise 4: Large Intestine Examination

Instructions: The large intestine is frequently examined radiographically after the introduction of a suitable contrast medium. This type of examination is called the barium enema (BE). This exercise pertains to the procedures and radiographs used for the two methods of barium enemas. Identify structures, fill in missing words, provide a short answer, match columns, select from a list, or choose true or false (explaining any statement you believe to be false) for each item.

1. What are the two basic methods of performing a barium enema?

    a. Oral and double-contrast
    b. Oral and enteroclysis (intubation)
    c. Single-contrast and double-contrast
    d Single-contrast and enteroclysis (intubation)

2. What is the most common type of contrast medium used for a BE?

    _____

3. Why should a high-density barium product be used as the contrast medium for double-contrast studies?

4. What two radiolucent contrast media can be used during the double-contrast study?

_____

5. When might an orally administered, water-soluble, iodinated contrast medium be used in place of a barium sulfate mixture?

6. What should be included in the instructions generally given to a patient in preparation for a BE?

7. What is considered the most important aspect of patient preparation for the BE?

8. What should the temperature of the barium be when the administration of a warm barium solution is desirable?

_____

9. How could the patient be affected if the barium solution is too warm?

10. What should the temperature of the barium be when administering cold barium solution?

_____

11. What are the advantages of filling the large intestine with a cold barium solution?

12. List three instructions that can be given to the patient to help the patient retain the barium during the examination.

13. How far above the level of the anus should the BE bag be placed (on a IV stand)?
    a. 6 to 12 inches
    b. 12 to 18 inches
    c. 18 to 24 inches
    d. 24 to 30 inches

14. What is the maximum distance that the enema tip should be inserted into the patient?
    a. 2.5 to 3 inches
    b. 3.5 to 4 inches
    c. 4.5 to 5 inches
    d. 5.5 to 6 inches

15. The last BE radiograph that is usually taken is the

    _____ film.

Items 16 through 19 pertain to the *PA projection*. Examine Fig. 17-16 as you answer the following items.

Fig. 17-16 PA large intestine.

16. How should the patient be placed for the PA projection?

   a. Prone
   b. Supine
   c. Upright
   d. Lateral recumbent

17. To which level of the patient should the cassette be centered?

   a. T12
   b. L2
   c. Iliac crests
   d. Symphysis pubis

18. How should the central ray be directed for the PA projection?

   a. Perpendicularly
   b. Angled caudally
   c. Angled cephalically

19. Identify each lettered structure shown in Fig. 17-17.

  A. _____ (flexure)

  B. _____ (flexure)

  C. _____

  D. _____

  E. _____

  F. _____

  G. _____

  H. _____

Fig. 17-17 PA colon.

Items 20 through 25 pertain to the *PA axial projection.* Examine Fig. 17-18 as you answer the following items.

Fig. 17-18 PA axial large intestine.

20. Which area of the large intestine is best demonstrated with the PA axial projection?

    a. Iliocecal
    b. Superior
    c. Rectosigmoid

21. How should the central ray be directed for the PA axial projection?

    a. Perpendicularly
    b. Angled caudally
    c. Angled cephalically

22. To which level of the patient should the central ray be directed for the PA axial projection?

    a. L2
    b. Symphysis pubis
    c. Anterior superior iliac spines

23. For the PA axial projection, which plane of the body should be centered to the midline of the table?

    a. Transverse
    b. Midsagittal
    c. Midcoronal

24. True or False. Both colic flexures should be seen with the PA axial projection.

25. Identify each lettered structure shown in Fig. 17-19.

    A. _____ (flexure)

    B. _____

    C. _____

    D. _____

Fig. 17-19 PA axial large intestine.

Items 26 through 30 pertain to the *PA oblique projection, RAO position*. Examine Fig. 17-20 as you answer the following items.

Fig. 17-20 PA oblique large intestine, RAO position.

26. True or False. For the right PA oblique projection (RAO position), the central ray should be directed 35 to 45 degrees caudally.

27. True or False. For the right PA oblique projection (RAO position), the patient should be rotated 35 to 45 degrees from the prone position.

28. True or False. Both colic flexures should be seen in the RAO position radiograph.

29. True or False. The right PA oblique projection (RAO position) is performed primarily to demonstrate the right colic flexure.

30. Identify each lettered structure shown in Fig. 17-21.

A. _____ (flexure)

B. _____ (flexure)

C. _____

D. _____

E. _____

Fig. 17-21 PA oblique large intestine, RAO position.

Items 31 through 33 pertain to the *PA oblique projection, LAO position.* Examine Fig. 17-22 as you answer the following items.

Fig. 17-22 PA oblique large intestine, LAO position.

31. To which level of the patient should the cassette be centered for the left PA oblique projection (LAO position)?
    a. T12
    b. L2
    c. Iliac crests
    d. Symphysis pubis

32. Which two structures of the large intestine are demonstrated primarily with the left PA oblique projection (LAO position)?
    a. Left colic flexure and ascending colon
    b. Left colic flexure and descending colon
    c. Right colic flexure and ascending colon
    d. Right colic flexure and descending colon

33. Identify each lettered structure shown in Fig. 17-23.

    A. _____ (flexure)

    B. _____ (flexure)

    C. _____

    D. _____

    E. _____

    F. _____

    G. _____

Fig. 17-23 PA oblique large intestine, LAO position.

Items 34 through 38 pertain to the *lateral projection*. Examine Fig. 17-24 as you answer the following items.

Fig. 17-24 Left lateral rectum.

34. For the lateral projection, to what level of the patient should a cassette that is 24 × 30 cm (10 × 12 in) be centered?

35. In the image of the left lateral projection, how is it determined that the patient was not rotated?

36. Which portions of the large intestine are of prime interest with the lateral projection?

    a. Sigmoid and rectum
    b. Cecum and ascending colon
    b. Left colic flexure and descending colon
    c. Right colic flexure and ascending colon

37. For the lateral projection, which plane of the body should be centered to the midline of the table?

    a. Transverse
    b. Midsagittal
    c. Midcoronal

38. Identify each lettered structure shown in Fig. 17-25.

    A. _____

    B. _____

    C. _____

    D. _____

Fig. 17-25 Left lateral rectum.

Items 39 through 43 pertain to the *AP projection.* Examine Fig. 17-26 as you answer the following items.

Fig. 17-26 AP large intestine.

39. Which plane of the body should be centered to the grid for the AP projection?

_____

40. To what level of the patient should the cassette be centered?

_____

41. True or False. The patient should suspend respiration for the exposure.

42. True or False. The entire colon should be demonstrated for the AP projection.

43. Identify each lettered structure shown in Fig. 17-27.

A. _____ (flexure)

B. _____

C. _____ (flexure)

D. _____

E. _____

F. _____

Fig. 17-27 AP large intestine.

Items 44 through 48 pertain to the *AP axial projection.* Examine Fig. 17-28 as you answer the following items.

Fig. 17-28 AP axial large intestine.

44. Which projection produces an image similar to the AP axial projection?

   a. AP projection
   b. PA axial projection
   c. Left PA oblique projection, LAO position
   d. Right PA oblique projection, RAO position

45. In which direction and how many degrees should the central ray be directed?

   a. Caudally 10 to 20 degrees
   b. Caudally 30 to 40 degrees
   c. Cephalically 10 to 20 degrees
   d. Cephalically 30 to 40 degrees

46. For the AP axial projection, where on the patient's anterior surface should the central ray enter when a cassette that is 35 × 43 cm (14 × 17 in) is used?

47. To produce a coned-down image of the AP axial projection on a cassette that is 24 × 30 cm (10 × 12 in), where on the patient should the central ray enter?

48. Identify each lettered structure shown in Fig. 17-29.

   A. _____

   B. _____

   C. _____

Fig. 17-29 AP axial large intestine.

Items 49 through 53 pertain to the *AP oblique projection, LPO position.* Examine Fig. 17-30 as you answer the following items.

Fig. 17-30 AP oblique large intestine, LPO position.

49. The left AP oblique projection (LPO position) produces an

   image similar to _____ projections

   (_____ position).

50. For the left AP oblique projection (LPO position), the pa-

   tient should be rotated _____ to _____ degrees.

51. For the left AP oblique projection (LPO position), which side of the patient—right or left—should be elevated away from the x-ray table?

   _____

52. Which flexure—right colic or left colic—should be well demonstrated with the left AP oblique projection (LPO position)?

   _____

53. Identify each lettered structure shown in Fig. 17-31.

   A. _____ (flexure)

   A. _____ (flexure)

   C. _____

   D. _____

   E. _____

   F. _____

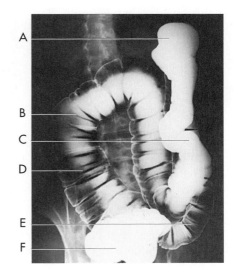

Fig. 17-31 AP oblique large intestine, LPO position.

Items 54 through 57 pertain to the *AP oblique projection (right posterior oblique [RPO] position)*. Examine Fig. 17-32 as you answer the following items.

Fig. 17-32 AP oblique large intestine, RPO position.

54. What other oblique position produces an image similar to the right AP oblique projection (RPO position)?

_____

55. Which flexure—right colic or left colic—should be well demonstrated with the right AP oblique projection (RPO position)?

_____

56. How many degrees should the patient be rotated from the supine position for the right AP oblique projection (RPO position)?

_____

57. Identify each lettered structure shown in Fig. 17-33.

A. _____ (flexure)

B. _____

C. _____ (flexure)

D. _____

E. _____

F. _____

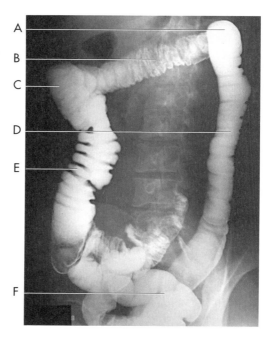

Fig. 17-33 AP oblique large intestine, RPO position.

Items 58 through 64 pertain to *AP or PA projections, right and left lateral decubitus positions.* Examine Figs. 17-34 and 17-35 as you answer the following items.

Fig. 17-34 AP large intestine, right lateral decubitus position.

Fig. 17-35 PA large intestine, left lateral decubitus position.

58. Which BE projection requires that the patient be placed in the right lateral recumbent position and that a horizontal central ray be directed to the midline of the patient at the level of the iliac crests?

    a. Right lateral

    b. AP, right lateral decubitus position

    c. Right AP oblique (RPO position)

    d. Right PA oblique (RAO position)

59. For lateral decubitus positions, what should be accomplished to ensure that the dependent side of the patient is demonstrated?

60. How much of the colon should be demonstrated in the image of a lateral decubitus position?

61. Name the lateral decubitus position that best demonstrates each of the following intestinal structures.

    a. Left colic flexure: _____

    b. Right colic flexure: _____

62. Figs. 17-36 and 17-37 are lateral decubitus radiographs. Examine the images and answer the questions that follow.

Left colic flexure

Sigmoid

Transverse colon

Right colic flexure

Fig. 17-36 Radiograph of the large intestine, lateral decubitus position.

Right colic flexure

Ascending colon

Rectum

Sigmoid

Descending colon

Left colic flexure

Fig. 17-37 Radiograph of the large intestine, lateral decubitus position.

a. Which image shows the left lateral decubitus position?

_____

b. Which image shows the right lateral decubitus position?

_____

c. Which image best demonstrates the left colic flexure?

_____

d. Which image best demonstrates the right colic flexure?

_____

e. Which image requires that the patient be placed in the left lateral recumbent position?

_____

f. Which image requires that the patient be placed in the right lateral recumbent position?

_____

Questions 63 and 64 pertain to BE radiographs performed with the patient in the upright position.

63. For upright frontal, oblique, and lateral projections, how is the centering of the cassette adjusted from that used for the recumbent positions? Why is this compensation necessary?

64. Examine Fig. 17-38 and answer the questions that follow.

Fig. 17-38 AP large intestine.

a. What body position was used to make this radiograph?

_____

b. What image characteristics led you to that conclusion?

65. Figs. 17-39 through 17-46 represent different projections used to obtain BE radiographs. Examine the images, then match the figures in Column A with the positions in Column B.

Fig. 17-39 BE radiograph.

Fig. 17-41 BE radiograph.

Fig. 17-40 BE radiograph.

Fig. 17-42 BE radiograph.

Fig. 17-43 BE radiograph.

Fig. 17-45 BE radiograph.

Fig. 17-44 BE radiograph.

Fig. 17-46 BE radiograph.

Column A		Column B
____	1. Fig. 17-39	a. LAO position
____	2. Fig. 17-40	b. LPO position
____	3. Fig. 17-41	c. AP axial position
____	4. Fig. 17-42	d. PA upright position
____	5. Fig. 17-43	e. AP recumbent position
____	6. Fig. 17-44	f. Left lateral position
____	7. Fig. 17-45	g. Postevacuation
____	8. Fig. 17-46	h. Lateral decubitus position

Self-Test: Anatomy and Positioning of the Alimentary Canal

Instructions: Answer the following questions by selecting the best choice.

1. In which body habitus type is the stomach almost horizontal and high in the abdomen?
   a. Sthenic
   b. Asthenic
   c. Hyposthenic
   d. Hypersthenic

2. Which curvature is located on the right (medial) border of the stomach?
   a. Lesser
   b. Greater
   c. Inferior
   d. Superior

3. Which area is the most superior part of the stomach?
   a. Head
   b. Body
   c. Fundus
   d. Pylorus

4. Which area is the most inferior part of the stomach?
   a. Body
   b. Cardia
   c. Fundus
   d. Pylorus

5. The distal esophagus empties its contents into which of the following:
   a. Duodenum
   b. Pyloric canal
   c. Duodenal bulb
   d. Cardiac antrum

6. Which opening is located between the stomach and small intestine?
   a. Cardiac orifice
   b. Pyloric orifice
   c. Ileocecal orifice
   d. Ampulla of Vater

7. Which opening is at the distal end of the small intestine?
   a. Anus
   b. Cardiac orifice
   c. Pyloric orifice
   d. Ileocecal orifice

8. Which structure is the proximal part of the small intestine?
   a. Ileum
   b. Pylorus
   c. Jejunum
   d. Duodenum

9. Which structure is the distal part of the small intestine?
   a. Ileum
   b. Cecum
   c. Jejunum
   d. Duodenum

10. In which abdominal region does the large intestine originate?
    a. Left iliac
    b. Right iliac
    c. Left lumbar
    d. Right lumbar

11. Which structure is the proximal part of the large intestine?
    a. Ileum
    b. Cecum
    c. Rectum
    d. Sigmoid

12. Which part of the large intestine is located between the ascending and descending parts of the colon?
    a. Cecum
    b. Rectum
    c. Sigmoid
    d. Transverse colon

13. Which structure is located between the ascending colon and the transverse colon?
    a. Sigmoid
    b. Left colic flexure
    c. Right colic flexure
    d. Descending colon

14. Where in the large intestine is the left colic flexure located?
    a. Between the cecum and the ascending colon
    b. Between the ascending colon and the transverse colon
    c. Between the transverse colon and the descending colon
    d. Between the descending colon and the sigmoid

15. Which structure is the pouch-like part of the large intestine situated below the junction of the ileum and the colon?
    a. Cecum
    b. Rectum
    c. Sigmoid
    d. Veriform appendix

16. Where in the large intestine is the sigmoid located?
    a. Between the cecum and the transverse colon
    b. Between the ascending colon and the transverse colon
    c. Between the descending colon and the rectum
    d. Between the transverse colon and the descending colon

17. Approximately how long does it usually take a barium meal to reach the ileocecal valve?
    a. 30 minutes to 1 hour
    b. 2 to 3 hours
    c. 4 to 5 hours
    d. 24 hours

18. Approximately how long does it usually take a barium meal to reach the rectum?
    a. 2 to 3 hours
    b. 4 to 5 hours
    c. 6 to 8 hours
    d. 24 hours

19. Which two imaging modalities are most commonly used to examine the alimentary canal after the introduction of a barium product?
    a. Fluoroscopy and sonography
    b. Fluoroscopy and radiography
    c. Computed tomography and sonography
    d. Computed tomography and radiography

20. Which type of contrast medium is most commonly used for examining the upper GI tract?
    a. An oily, viscous compound
    b. A barium sulfate suspension
    c. A nonionic injectable compound
    d. A water-soluble, iodinated solution

21. To best demonstrate the swallowing function, in which position should the patient be placed to begin the fluoroscopic phase of single-contrast examinations of the esophagus?
    a. Upright
    b. Left lateral decubitus
    c. Recumbent LAO
    d. Recumbent RPO

22. Which two recumbent oblique positions can be used to best demonstrate an unobstructed image of a barium-filled esophagus between the vertebrae and the heart?
    a. LAO and LPO
    b. LAO and RPO
    c. RAO and LPO
    d. RAO and RPO

23. Which of the following is a major advantage of the double-contrast UGI examination over the single-contrast UGI examination?
    a. The patient can better tolerate the procedure.
    b. Radiation exposure to the patient is reduced.
    c. Small lesions on the mucosal lining are better demonstrated.
    d. The examination can be performed with the patient upright instead of recumbent

24. Which description refers to the biphasic GI examination?
    a. A single-contrast study of the entire alimentary canal
    b. A single-contrast study of the upper GI tract
    c. A double-contrast study of the upper GI tract
    d. A combination single-contrast and double-contrast study of the upper GI tract

25. Which body habitus produces the greatest visceral movement when a patient is moved from the prone position to the upright position?
    a. Sthenic
    b. Asthenic
    c. Hyposthenic
    d. Hypersthenic

26. For the double-contrast UGI examination, which projection produces the best image of a gas-filled duodenal bulb and pyloric canal?
    a. Left AP oblique projection (LPO position) with the patient upright
    b. Left AP oblique projection (LPO position) with the patient recumbent
    c. Right PA oblique projection (RAO position) with the patient upright
    d. Right PA oblique projection (RAO position) with the patient recumbent

27. For the single-contrast UGI examination with the patient recumbent, which projection produces the best image of a barium-filled duodenal bulb and pyloric canal?
    a. AP projection
    b. Left lateral projection
    c. Left AP oblique projection (LPO position)
    d. Right PA oblique projection (RAO position)

28. For the UGI examination with the patient recumbent, which projection best stimulates gastric peristalsis to better demonstrate the pyloric canal and duodenal bulb?
    a. AP projection
    b. Left lateral projection
    c. Left AP oblique projection (LPO position)
    d. Right PA oblique projection (RAO position)

29. Which breathing procedure should be performed by the patient when UGI radiographs are exposed?

   a. Slow, deep breathing
   b. Quick, panting breaths
   c. Suspended expiration
   d. Suspended inspiration

30. For the double-contrast UGI examination with the patient recumbent, which projection produces the best image of a gas-filled fundus?

   a. Left lateral projection
   b. AP projection, left lateral decubitus position
   c. Left AP oblique projection (LPO position)
   d. Right PA oblique projection (RAO position)

31. For the UGI examination with the patient recumbent, which projection best demonstrates the right retrogastric space?

   a. Right lateral projection
   b. AP projection, right lateral decubitus position
   c. Left AP oblique projection (LPO position)
   d. Right PA oblique projection (RAO position)

32. For the AP projection with the patient supine (as part of the UGI examination), which procedure should be performed to best demonstrate a diaphragmatic herniation (hiatal hernia)?

   a. Angle the central ray 30 to 35 degrees caudally.
   b. Tilt the table and patient into a full Trendelenburg position.
   c. Instruct the patient to suspend respiration after full inspiration.
   d. Place radiolucent cushions under the thorax to elevate the shoulders.

33. To which level of the patient should the central ray be directed for the right PA oblique projection (RAO position) as part of the UGI examination?

   a. T10
   b. T12
   c. L2
   d. L4

34. Which examination of the alimentary canal requires that a series of radiographs be taken at specific time intervals after the ingestion of the contrast medium?

   a. BE
   b. Esophagography
   c. Small bowel series
   d. UGI series

35. For a small bowel series of a patient with hypomotility of the small intestine, which procedure should be performed to accelerate peristalsis?

   a. Roll the patient 360 degrees.
   b. Instruct the patient to drink a glass of ice water.
   c. Instruct the patient to perform the Valsalva maneuver.
   d. Tilt the table and patient into a full Trendelenburg position.

36. The visualization of which structure usually indicates the completion of a small bowel series?

   a. Ileum
   b. Cecum
   c. Jejunum
   d. Duodenum

37. Which procedure should be used during a BE to relax the large intestine and enable the patient to better retain the barium sulfate suspension?

   a. Instruct the patient to perform the Valsalva maneuver.
   b. Raise the barium bag to 24 inches above the rectum.
   c. Administer cold (41° F) barium sulfate suspension.
   d. Administer warm (95° F) barium sulfate suspension.

38. Which procedure should be performed when the enema tip is inserted during a BE?

   a. Lubricate the tip with petroleum jelly.
   b. Place the patient in the Trendelenburg position.
   c. Inflate the air-filled retention tip before insertion.
   d. Ensure that the tip is inserted 2 to 4 inches (5 to 10 cm).

39. Before the enema tip is inserted during a BE, why should a small amount of barium sulfate mixture be allowed to run into a waste basket?

   a. To lubricate the enema tip
   b. To remove air from the tube
   c. To determine if the mixture is too warm or too cold
   d. To ensure that the consistency of the mixture is adequate

40. For the PA projection during a BE, what is the advantage of placing the x-ray table and patient in a slight Trendelenburg position?

   a. To demonstrate the ileocecal valve
   b. To enable more air to be injected into the colon
   c. To help separate overlapping loops of distal bowel
   d. To move the transverse colon higher in the abdomen

41. Which structures of the large intestine are of primary interest with AP axial or PA axial projections during a BE?

   a. Sigmoid and rectum
   b. Cecum and ileocecal valve
   c. Left and right colic flexures
   d. Ascending and descending colons

42. How many degrees and in which direction should the central ray be directed for the PA axial projection during a BE?

    a. 20 to 25 degrees caudad
    b. 20 to 25 degrees cephalad
    c. 30 to 40 degrees caudad
    d. 30 to 40 degrees cephalad

43. Which structure of the large intestine is of primary interest for the right PA oblique projection (RAO position) during BE examinations?

    a. Anal canal
    b. Left colic flexure
    c. Right colic flexure
    d. Descending colon

44. Which two oblique projections can be performed to best demonstrate the left colic flexure during a BE?

    a. Left PA oblique projection (LAO position) and left AP oblique projection (LPO position)
    b. Left PA oblique projection (LAO position) and right AP oblique projection (RPO position)
    c. Right PA oblique projection (RAO position) and left AP oblique projection (LPO position)
    d. Right PA oblique projection (RAO position) and right AP oblique projection (RPO position)

45. Which structure of the large intestine is best demonstrated if the patient is rotated 45 degrees from a supine position to move the left side of the abdomen away from the x-ray table during a BE?

    a. Ileum
    b. Cecum
    c. Left colic flexure
    d. Right colic flexure

46. For the right lateral decubitus position as part of a barium enema, which procedure should be done to ensure that the ascending colon is demonstrated in the image?

    a. Center the cassette to the iliac crests.
    b. Elevate the patient on a radiolucent support.
    c. Tilt the table and patient into a full Trendelenburg position.
    d. Make the exposure after the patient suspends respiration.

47. What is the proper sequence for filling the large intestine with barium when performing a BE?

    a. Rectum, sigmoid, ascending colon, transverse colon, and descending colon
    b. Rectum, sigmoid, descending colon, transverse colon, and ascending colon
    c. Sigmoid, rectum, ascending colon, transverse colon, and descending colon
    d. Sigmoid, rectum, descending colon, transverse colon, and ascending colon

48. Which BE projection requires that a 24 × 30 cm (10 × 12 in) cassette be centered lengthwise approximately 2 to 3 inches (5 to 7.5 cm) above the level of the symphysis pubis in the midcoronal plane?

    a. AP projection
    b. Lateral projection
    c. AP projection, left lateral decubitus position
    d. Left AP oblique projection (LPO position)

49. Which BE projection usually does not require that both flexures be included in the image?

    a. AP projection
    b. Lateral projection
    c. AP projection, lateral decubitus position
    d. Right PA oblique projection (RAO position)

50. For the PA projection as part of the UGI examination, why should the lower lung fields be included on a 35 × 43 cm (14 × 17 in) cassette?

    a. To demonstrate pneumothorax
    b. To demonstrate a possible hiatal hernia
    c. To demonstrate fluid levels in the thorax
    d. To demonstrate the gas bubble in the fundus of the stomach

If your school has access to Mosby's Radiographic Instructional Series on Anatomy, Positioning, and Procedures, review Unit 17 at this time. Your instructor may request that you respond to the series' exercises on paper. This unit covers the following essential projections:

Esophagus
AP or PA projections
PA oblique projections, RAO or LPO
Lateral projections, right or left

Stomach and duodenum
PA projections
PA oblique projections, RAO
AP oblique projections, LPO
Lateral projections, right only
AP projections

Small intestine
PA or AP projections

Large intestine
PA projections
PA axial projections
PA oblique projections, RAO
PA oblique, projections LAO
Lateral projections, right or left
AP projections
AP axial projections
AP oblique projections, LPO
AP oblique projections, RPO
AP or PA projections, right lateral decubitus
PA or AP projections, left lateral decubitus
AP, PA, oblique, or lateral projections: upright

CHAPTER 18

Urinary System

SECTION 1

Anatomy of the Urinary System

Exercise 1

Instructions: This exercise pertains to urinary structures. Identify structures for each question.

1. Identify each lettered structure shown in Fig. 18-1.

   A. _____

   B. _____

   C. _____

   D. _____

   E. _____

   F. _____

2. Identify each lettered structure shown in Fig. 18-2.

   A. _____

   B. _____

   C. _____

   D. _____

   E. _____

   F. _____

Fig. 18-1 Anterior aspect of the urinary system in relation to the surrounding structures.

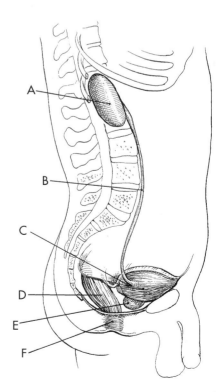

Fig. 18-2 Lateral aspect of the male urinary system in relation to the surrounding structures.

3. Identify each lettered part of the kidney shown in Fig. 18-3.

A. _____

B. _____

C. _____

D. _____

E. _____

F. _____

G. _____

H. _____

I. _____

Fig. 18-3 Midcoronal section of a kidney.

4. Identify each lettered structure shown in Fig. 18-4.

A. _____

B. _____

C. _____

D. _____

E. _____

F. _____

G. _____

H. _____

I. _____

J. _____

K. _____

5. Identify each lettered structure shown in Fig. 18-5.

A. _____

B. _____

C. _____

D. _____

E. _____

F. _____

G. _____

H. _____

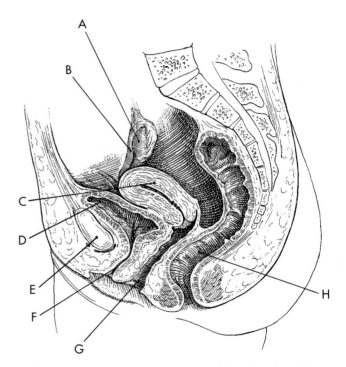

Fig. 18-5 Midsagittal section through the female pelvis.

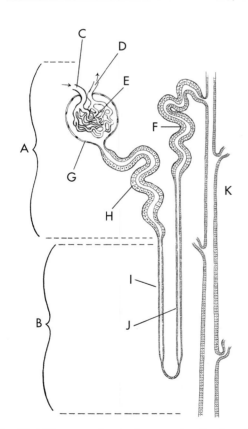

Fig. 18-4 Diagram of a nephron and collecting duct.

6. Identify each lettered structure shown in Fig. 18-6.

A. _____   D. _____

B. _____   E. _____

C. _____   F. _____

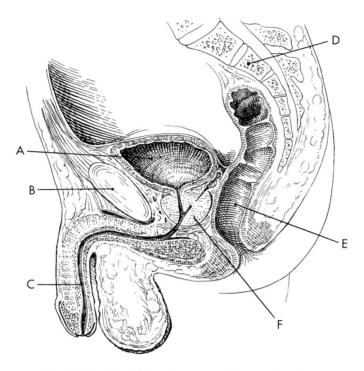

Fig. 18-6 Midsagittal section through the male pelvis.

Exercise 2

Instructions: Use the following clues to complete the cross-word puzzle below. All answers refer to the urinary system.

ACROSS

3. Outer renal tissue
4. This arteriole leaves the capsule
6. Filtrate derivative
7. Another term for suprarenal
8. Urine vessel from glomerular capsule
10. Cup-shaped urine receivers
12. Cone-shaped renal segments
15. Cluster of blood vessels
16. Urinary reservoir
17. Functional renal unit
18. Musculomembranous excretory duct
19. Medial opening of a kidney

DOWN

1. This arteriole enters the capsule
2. Inner renal tissue
3. Membranous cup; Bowman's _____
5. Central renal cavity
6. External excretory tube
9. Male gland
11. Gland that is found on a kidney
13. Glomerular fluid
14. Primary organ of urinary system

Exercise 3

Instructions: This exercise pertains to the anatomy of the urinary system. Fill in missing words for each question.

1. The kidneys and ureters are part of the

   _____ system.

2. The organ that removes waste products from the blood is

   the _____.

3. The gland that sits on the superior pole of each kidney is

   the _____ gland.

4. Blood vessels, nerves, and the ureter enter a kidney
   through an opening known as the

   _____.

5. The hilum is located on the _____
   border of the kidney.

6. In the average (sthenic) person, the superior pole of the

   kidney is located at the _____ vertebral level.

7. The microscopic functional unit of the kidney is the

   _____.

8. Nephron units are found in the layer of renal tissue known

   as the _____.

9. The proximal portion of a nephron consisting of a double-

   walled membranous cup is the _____
   capsule.

10. A cluster of blood capillaries surrounded by a Bowman's

    capsule is a _____.

11. A glomerulus branches off the _____
    artery.

12. The blood vessel entering a glomerular capsule is the

    _____ arteriole; the blood vessel
    leaving a glomerular capsule is the

    _____ arteriole.

13. The fluid that passes from the glomerulus to the glomerular capsule is _____

    _____.

14. Urine from collecting ducts drains into minor

    _____.

15. Minor calyces drain urine into major

    _____.

16. Major calyces unite to form the expanded, funnel-shaped

    renal _____.

17. The long tubes that transport urine from the kidneys are the

    _____.

18. Ureters transport urine from kidneys to the

    _____ _____.

19. The musculomembranous tube that conveys urine from
    the urinary bladder to outside the body is the

    _____.

20. The gland that surrounds the proximal part of the male urethra is the _____.

Exercise 4: Venipuncture and IV Contrast Media Administration

Instructions: This exercise pertains to venipuncture and IV contrast media administration. Items require you to write a short answer or select from a list.

1. Which condition should be prevented if strict aseptic techniques are used when administering medications intravenously?

   a. The patient lapsing into shock
   b. Introducing infection into the patient
   c. Injecting an excessive amount of medication

2. How does the use of an IV filter affect a bolus injection?

   a. The rate of injection will be reduced.
   b. The introduction of foreign matter will increase.
   c. The time required to inject the medication will be reduced.

3. What are the three parts of a syringe?

   a. Tip, barrel, and bevel
   b. Tip, barrel, and plunger
   c. Hub, cannula, and bevel
   d. Hub, cannula, and plunger

4. What are the three parts of a hypodermic needle?

   a. Tip, barrel, and bevel
   b. Tip, barrel, and plunger
   c. Hub, cannula, and bevel
   d. Hub, cannula, and plunger

5. What does the term *needle gauge* refer to?

   a. The angle of the bevel
   b. The length of the needle
   c. The diameter of the needle

6. What injection apparatus is preferred for most IV administrations?

   a. Butterfly set
   b. Over-the-needle cannula
   c. Seldinger-technique needle

7. What procedure should be performed to maintain a closed system with a multiple-dose vial of medication?

8. When assessing vessels for venipuncture, why should a vessel *not* be used if a pulse is detected?

9. From the list below, circle the four sites that are most often used for establishing IV access.

   a. Anterior hand
   b. Posterior hand
   c. Femoral artery
   d. Anterior forearm
   e. Posterior forearm
   f. Ulnar aspect of the wrist
   g. Radial aspect of the wrist
   h. Anterior aspect of the elbow

10. Describe how the skin should be prepared before inserting a needle into a vein.

11. How far above the site of a venipuncture should the tourniquet be placed?

    _____

12. How should the IV needle be inserted—bevel-up or bevel-down?

    _____

13. When inserting an IV needle into the patient, what angle should exist between the needle and the patient's skin surface?

    _____

14. What is the significance of a backflow of blood into the syringe during a venipuncture procedure?

15. What procedure should a radiographer perform if both walls of the vein have been punctured by the needle?

16. What is infiltration?
    a. The procedure for using an IV filter in tubing
    b. The introduction of a hypodermic needle into a vein
    c. The process of injecting fluid into tissues instead of a vein

17. Which other term refers to infiltration?
    a. Extraction
    b. Extirpation
    c. Extravasation

18. Which procedure should a radiographer perform *after* a needle has been removed from a vein?
    a. Apply a tourniquet 3 to 4 inches above the puncture site.
    b. Using a 2 × 2 pad of gauze, apply pressure directly to the injection site.
    c. Clean the area using a circular motion covering an area that is approximately 2 inches in diameter.

19. From the list below, circle the four symptoms that may indicate the occurence of infiltration.
    a. Pain
    b. Burning
    c. Redness
    d. Swelling
    e. Dyspnea
    f. Sneezing
    g. Rapid pulse
    h. Hypotension

20. From the list below, circle the five golden rules of medication administration.
    a. The right time
    b. The right route
    c. The right patient
    d. The right syringe
    e. The right amount
    f. The right medication
    g. The right technologist
    h. The right body position

SECTION 2

Positioning of the Urinary System

Exercise 1: Excretory Urography

Instructions: Radiography of the urinary system comprises numerous specialized procedures. The most common radiographic examination of the urinary system is the excretory urogram. This exercise pertains to excretory urography. Identify structures, fill in missing words, select from a list, provide a short answer, or choose true or false (explain any item you believe to be false) for each question.

Questions 1 through 22 pertain to general information concerning excretory urography.

1. The radiographic investigation of the renal drainage system is accomplished by various procedures classified under the general term of _____.

2. Which two terms refer to the excretory urogram examination?
   a. Cystourethrography and retrograde urography
   b. Cystourethrography and intravenous pyelography
   c. Intravenous urography and retrograde urography
   d. Intravenous urography and intravenous pyelography

3. From the list below, circle four terms that identify the typical contrast media currently used in excretory urography.
   a. Ionic
   b. Nonionic
   c. Iodinated
   d. Noniodinated
   e. Injectable
   f. Noninjectable

4. From the list below, circle the mild adverse reactions to iodinated contrast medium administration.
   a. Hives
   b. Death
   c. Nausea
   d. Dyspnea
   e. Vomiting
   f. Warm feeling
   g. Cardiac arrest
   h. Renal shutdown
   i. Flush appearance
   j. Respiratory arrest
   k. Edema of the respiratory mucous membranes

5. How soon after the injection of a contrast medium are symptoms of a reaction most likely to occur?
   a. Within 5 minutes
   b. Between 5 to 10 minutes
   c. More than 10 minutes

6. From the list below, circle the four typical procedures that a patient might ideally experience when preparing for the intravenous urography (IVU) examination.
   a. Laxative
   b. Cleansing enema
   c. Light evening meal
   d. Liquid diet for 3 to 4 days
   e. Low-residue diet for 1 or 2 days
   f. Drinking 32 ounces of water to fill the bladder
   g. NPO after midnight on the day of the examination

7. What is the purpose of giving a child 12 ounces of carbonated beverage just before the start of IVU?

8. Why should an immobilization band *not* be applied across the patient's upper abdomen in an effort to control motion during IVU?

9. What is the purpose of applying compression over the distal ends of the ureters?

10. Where on the abdomen should compression pads be located to compress the ureters?

11. When ureteral compression is used, why should the pressure be slowly released when the compression device is no longer needed?

12. Why is ureteral compression currently *not* often used in excretory urography?

13. Why might an upright AP projection be made of the abdomen before the inejction of the contrast medium?

14. What identification data should be included on every postinjection radiograph?

15. Why is it desirable to have the patient remove his or her underwear?

16. Why should the patient be instructed to empty his or her bladder just before IVU is to begin?

    a. To locate the ureteral openings
    b. To measure the capacity of the bladder
    c. To prevent dilution of the opacified urine

17. From the list below, circle the five reasons that AP projections with the patient recumbent are performed as the scout radiograph.

    a. To demonstrate the bladder
    b. To identify the location of the kidneys
    c. To demonstrate the presence of calculi
    d. To demonstrate the contour of the kidneys
    e. To check the radiographic exposure factors
    f. To demonstrate the mobility of the kidneys
    g. To examine for radiopaque artifacts on the positioning table
    h. To determine how well the patient's gastrointestinal (GI) tract was cleaned

18. What can be done to enhance the filling of renal structures with contrast medium when the patient is supine?

    a. Place supports under the patient's knees.
    b. Place a support under the patient's lumbar region.
    c. Direct the central ray 20 to 25 degrees caudally.
    d. Tilt the x-ray table and patient to the Trendelenburg position.

19. Approximately how long after a bolus injection of the contrast medium should the exposure be made to best demonstrate a nephrogram?

    a. 30 seconds
    b. 3 minutes
    c. 5 minutes

20. How long after the completion of the contrast medium injection does the contrast agent usually begin to appear in the renal pelvis?

    a. 30 seconds to 1 minute
    b. 2 to 8 minutes
    c. 10 to 14 minutes
    d. 15 to 20 minutes

21. How long after the injection of the contrast medium does the greatest concentration usually appear within the kidneys?

    a. 30 seconds to 1 minute
    b. 2 to 8 minutes
    c. 15 to 20 minutes
    d. 30 to 45 minutes

22. A postvoiding radiograph is usually the last radiograph taken to demonstrate which structure(s)?

    a. Ureters
    b. Bladder
    c. Kidneys

Items 23 through 32 pertain to the *AP projection.* Examine Fig. 18-7 as you answer the following items.

Fig. 18-7 Supine urogram, AP projection.

23. True or False. The AP projection may be obtained with the patient supine or upright.

24. True or False. Preliminary (scout) radiographs are most often obtained with the patient supine.

25. True or False. Postinjection radiographs are most often obtained with the patient upright.

26. What is the most likely purpose for obtaining an AP projection radiograph with the patient standing?

    a. To elongate the ureters
    b. To demonstrate ureteral reflux
    c. To demonstrate air-fluid levels
    d. To demonstrate the mobility of the kidneys

27. What adjustment in the supine patient's position can be made to help demonstrate the distal ends of the ureters?

    a. Place supports under the patient's knees.
    b. Place a support under the patient's lumbar region.
    c. Position a compression band around the patient's abdomen.
    d. Tilt the table and patient 15 to 20 degrees Trendelenburg.

28. Which procedure should be performed if the bladder is not seen in the AP projection to demonstrate the entire urinary system?

    a. Center the cassette to the level of L3.
    b. Direct the central ray 10 to 15 degrees cephalically.
    c. Tilt the table and patient 10 to 15 degrees Trendelenburg.
    d. Make a separate AP projection radiograph of the bladder.

29. What should be done to reduce the lordotic curvature when performing the AP projection with the patient recumbent?

    a. Place supports under the patient's knees.
    b. Position a compression band around the patient's abdomen.
    c. Tilt the table and patient 10 to 15 degrees Trendelenburg.

30. Why is it desirable to include the area below the pubic symphysis for older male patients?

    a. To demonstrate distal ureters
    b. To demonstrate ureteral reflux
    c. To demonstrate the prostate region
    d. To demonstrate urinary bladder calculi

31. If a device is used for ureteral compression, to which level of the patient should it be centered?

    a. L1 to L3
    b. At the level of the iliac crests
    c. 2 inches (5 cm) above the iliac crests
    d. 2 inches (5 cm) above the superior border of the pubic symphysis

32. Identify each lettered structure shown in Fig. 18-8.

A. _____

B. _____

C. _____

D. _____

E. _____

Fig. 18-8 AP projection of the urinary system.

Questions 33 through 38 pertain to *AP oblique projections.* Examine Fig. 18-9 as you answer the following questions.

Fig. 18-9 Urogram, AP oblique projection (RPO position).

33. Into which position should the patient be placed when beginning to position for either type of AP oblique projection?

   a. Prone
   b. Supine
   c. Lateral recumbent

34. When performing the AP oblique projection (RPO position), which kidney—left or right—will be parallel with the plane of the cassette?

   _____

35. Approximately how many degrees should the patient be rotated from the supine position to an oblique position to demonstrate renal and urinary structures?

   a. 10 degrees
   b. 20 degrees
   c. 30 degrees
   d. 40 degrees

36. Which structure should be centered to the grid for the AP oblique projection (LPO position)?

   a. Left kidney
   b. Right kidney
   c. Vertebral column

37. To which level of the patient should the cassette be centered?

    a. L3
    b. Iliac crests
    c. Anterior superior iliac crests
    d. Pubic symphysis

38. Where should the central ray enter the patient?

    a. 2 inches lateral to the midline on the elevated side
    b. 2 inches lateral to the midline on the dependent side
    c. Centered to the midline 2 inches below the iliac crests

Items 39 through 43 pertain to the lateral projection (lateral recumbent position). Examine Fig. 18-10 as you answer the following items.

Fig. 18-10 Urogram, lateral projection.

39. Which plane of the body should be centered to the grid?

_____

40. Describe how the patient's arms and hands should be placed?

41. Which areas of the patient should be examined to ensure that the patient is not rotated?

42. The exposure should be made at the end of

_____ (inspiration or expiration).

43. Exposure factors should produce a _____ (long or short) scale of contrast.

Items 44 through 50 pertain to the *lateral projection (dorsal decubitus position)*. Examine Fig. 18-11 as you answer the following items.

Fig. 18-11 Urogram, lateral projection (dorsal decubitus position).

44. The dorsal decubitus position requires that the patient be

    _____ (prone or supine).

45. The long axis of the cassette should be centered to the

    _____ plane.

46. Which area of the patient should be closest to the grid?
    a. Side
    b. Anterior
    c. Posterior

47. Which level of the patient should be centered to the cassette?
    a. L3
    b. Crests of the ilia
    c. Anterior superior iliac crests
    d. Pubic symphysis

48. True or False. Only male patients should have gonadal shielding for this type of projection.

49. True or False. The exposure should be made at the end of inspiration.

50. True or False. The central ray should be directed horizontal and perpendicular to the center of the cassette.

Exercise 2: Retrograde Urography

Instructions: Retrograde urography is a radiographic procedure that demonstrates certain urinary structures. This exercise pertains to retrograde urography. Provide a short answer, select from a list, or choose true or false (explaining any statement you believe to be false) for each item.

Examine Fig. 18-12 as you answer the following items about retrograde urography.

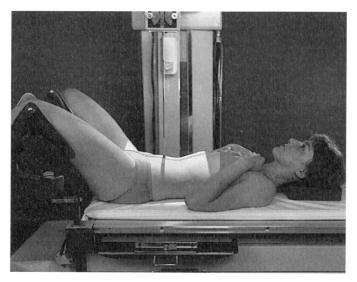

Fig. 18-12 Patient positioned on the table for retrograde urography.

1. True or False. Retrograde urography differs from excretory urography in that the contrast medium is injected directly into the kidney by means of a percutaneous injection through the skin.

2. True or False. Retrograde urography is performed on a regular x-ray table.

3. At the beginning of the retrograde urographic examination, the patient is placed in the modified _____ position.
   a. Prone
   b. Upright
   c. Lithotomy
   d. Lateral recumbent

4. Which cassette size should be used for urograms of the typical adult?
   a. 18 × 24 cm
   b. 24 × 30 cm
   c. 35 × 43 cm

5. Who should inject the contrast medium?
   a. Urologist
   b. Radiologist
   c. Radiographer

6. Describe how a kidney function test can be performed during retrograde urography.

7. List the three AP projection radiographs that usually comprise a retrograde urographic examination.

8. Why might the head of the x-ray table be lowered 10 to 15 degrees during the retrograde pyelography procedure?

9. Which retrograde urographic radiograph sometimes requires that the head of the table be elevated 35 to 40 degrees?
   a. Pyelogram
   b. Ureterogram
   c. Preliminary radiograph showing catheter insertion

10. After necessary AP projections are made, which oblique positions are often used for oblique projections?
   a. RPO and LPO
   b. RPO and LAO
   c. RAO and LPO
   d. RAO and LAO

Exercise 3: Retrograde Cystography

Instructions: Projections obtained during retrograde cystography often include an AP projection, both AP oblique projections (RPO and LPO positions), and a lateral projection. This exercise pertains to those projections. Fill in missing words or provide a short answer for each item.

1. Describe how the contrast medium is introduced into the patient for retrograde cystography.

Questions 2 through 11 pertain to *AP axial or PA axial projections*. Examine Fig. 18-13 as you answer the following questions.

Fig. 18-13 AP axial bladder.

2. For the typical adult, which size cassette should be used to demonstrate the bladder, and how should it be placed in the cassette holder?

   a. 18 × 24 cm; crosswise
   b. 18 × 24 cm; lengthwise
   c. 24 × 30 cm; crosswise
   d. 24 × 30 cm; lengthwise

3. Which structures are sometimes better demonstrated with the head of the table lowered 15 to 20 degrees?

   a. Prostate gland and urethra
   b. Lower (distal) ends of the ureters
   c. Upper (proximal) ends of the ureters

4. Why should patients in the supine position extend the lower limbs?

   a. To demonstrate ureteral reflux
   b. To retard the excretion of opacified urine from the bladder
   c. To enable the lumbar lordotic curve to arch the pelvis enough to tilt the pubic bones inferiorly

5. How many degrees and in which direction should the central ray be directed for the AP axial projection?

   a. 5 degrees caudad
   b. 5 degrees cephalad
   c. 15 degrees caudad
   d. 15 degrees cephalad

6. To which level of the patient should the central ray enter for the AP axial projection?

   a. The iliac crests
   b. 2 to 3 inches (5 to 7.5 cm) above the upper border of the pubic symphysis
   c. 2 to 3 inches (5 to 7.5 cm) below the upper border of the pubic symphysis

7. For the AP axial projection, to which level of the patient should the cassette be centered?

   a. The iliac crests
   b. 2 to 3 inches (5 to 7.5 cm) above the upper border of the pubic symphysis
   c. 2 to 3 inches (5 to 7.5 cm) below the upper border of the pubic symphysis

8. Which breathing instructions should be given to the patient?

   a. Slow breathing
   b. Suspend breathing after expiration
   c. Suspend breathing after inspiration

9. How should the patient be positioned to best demonstrate the prostate?

   a. Prone
   b. Supine
   c. Upright
   d. Lateral recumbent

10. How should the central ray be directed to best demonstrate the prostate?

    a. Caudally
    b. Cephalically
    c. Perpendicularly

11. How should the pubic bones be demonstrated in the image of the AP axial projection?

    a. They should superimpose both the bladder neck and the proximal urethra.
    b. They should be projected above both the bladder neck and the proximal urethra.
    c. They should be projected below both the bladder neck and the proximal urethra.

Items 12 through 16 pertain to *AP oblique projections*. Examine Fig. 18-14 as you answer the following items.

Fig. 18-14 Retrograde cystogram, AP oblique projection (RPO position).

12. In which position should the patient be placed?
    a. Semiprone
    b. Semisupine
    c. Lateral recumbent

13. How should the patient's uppermost thigh be positioned to prevent it from superimposing the bladder in AP oblique projections?
    a. Crossed over the other thigh
    b. Flexed and placed at right angles to the abdomen
    c. Extended and abducted enough to prevent its superimposition on the bladder area

14. How many degrees should the patient be rotated for AP oblique projections?
    a. 10 to 15
    b. 20 to 30
    c. 40 to 60

15. From the list below, circle the two ways that the central ray can be directed for AP oblique projections.
    a. Perpendicularly
    b. 10 degrees caudally
    c. 10 degrees cephalically
    d. 20 degrees caudally
    e. 20 degrees cephalically

16. The bladder neck should be seen

    _____ (above or below) the pubic bones.

Questions 17 through 20 pertain to the *lateral projection*. Examine Fig. 18-15 as you answer the following questions.

Fig. 18-15 Cystogram, lateral projection.

17. The patient should be placed in the

    _____ _____ position.

18. For lateral projections, the cassette should be centered to the patient at a level 2 to 3 inches (5 to 7.5 cm) above the

    _____ _____.

19. How should the central ray be directed?
    a. Horizontally
    b. Perpendicularly
    c. Angled caudally
    d. Angled cephalically

20. Which imaged structures can determine whether the patient was rotated from the lateral position?
    a. Lumbar vertebrae
    b. Crests of the ilia
    c. Hips and femora

Exercise 4: Male Cystourethrography

Instructions: This exercise pertains to male cystourethrography. Provide a short answer, select from a list, or choose true or false (explaining any statement you believe to be false) for each item.

1. Define *cystourethrography*.

2. Describe how the contrast medium is introduced into the urinary structures of interest.

3. After the contrast medium is introduced into the patient, in which two positions can the patient be placed to demonstrate urinary structures?
   a. RAO and LAO
   b. RAO and LPO
   c. RPO and LAO
   d. RPO and LPO

4. How many degrees should the patient be rotated for the desired oblique projection?
   a. 15 to 20 degrees
   b. 25 to 30 degrees
   c. 35 to 40 degrees

5. To which level of the patient should the cassette be centered?
   a. Crests of the ilia
   b. Anterior superior iliac spines
   c. 2 inches (5 cm) above the superior border of the pubic symphysis
   d. Superior border of the pubic symphysis

6. True or False. To ensure adequate coverage, the cassette should be placed lengthwise.

7. True or False. To ensure that the entire urethra is filled, the exposure should be made while the physician is injecting the contrast medium.

8. True or False. After the bladder is filled with contrast medium, the voiding film can be exposed with the patient in either a posterior oblique or upright position.

9. True or False. The radiation field should be large enough to include the entire urinary system on all radiographs.

10. True or False. The image of the urethra should be seen posterior to the superimposed pubic and ischial rami of the dependent side when the patient is properly rotated into a posterior oblique position.

Exercise 5: Identifying Urinary System Radiographs

Instructions: Identify each of the following radiographs by selecting the best choice from the list provided for each image.

1. Fig. 18-16:
   a. Excretory urogram, AP projection
   b. Retrograde urogram, AP projection
   c. Excretory cystogram, AP projection
   d. Preliminary (scout) radiograph, AP projection

Fig. 18-16 Urinary examination radiograph.

2. Fig. 18-17:

   a. Excretory urogram, AP projection
   b. Retrograde urogram, AP projection
   c. Excretory cystogram, AP projection
   d. Preliminary (scout) radiograph, AP projection

3. Fig. 18-18:

   a. Excretory urogram, AP projection
   b. Retrograde urogram, AP projection
   c. Excretory cystogram, AP projection
   d. Preliminary (scout) radiograph, AP projection

Fig. 18-17 Urinary examination radiograph.

Fig. 18-18 Urinary examination radiograph.

4. Fig. 18-19:
   a. Excretory urogram, AP oblique projection (LPO position)
   b. Excretory urogram, AP oblique projection (RPO position)
   c. Retrograde cystogram, AP oblique projection (LPO position)
   d. Retrograde cystogram, AP oblique projection (RPO position)

Fig. 18-19 Urinary examination radiograph.

5. Fig. 18-20:
   a. Urogram, lateral projection
   b. Urogram, left lateral decubitus
   c. Excretory urogram, AP oblique projection (RPO position)
   d. Excretory urogram, AP oblique projection (LPO position)

Fig. 18-20 Urinary examination radiograph.

6. Fig. 18-21:
   a. Prevoiding filled bladder, AP projection
   b. Postvoiding emptied bladder, AP projection
   c. Retrograde cystogram, AP oblique projection (RPO position)
   d. Injection cystouretrogram, AP oblique urethra (RPO position)

Fig. 18-21 Urinary examination radiograph.

7. Fig. 18-22:

   a. Prevoiding filled bladder, AP projection
   b. Postvoiding emptied bladder, AP projection
   c. Retrograde cystogram, AP oblique projection (RPO position)
   d. Injection cystouretrogram, AP oblique urethra (RPO position)

9. Fig. 18-24:

   a. Excretory cystogram, AP projection
   b. Retrograde cystogram, AP projection
   c. Postvoiding emptied bladder, AP projection
   d. Retrograde cystogram, AP oblique projection (RPO position)

Fig. 18-22 Urinary examination radiograph.

Fig. 18-24 Urinary examination radiograph.

8. Fig. 18-23:

   a. Excretory cystogram, AP projection
   b. Retrograde cystogram, AP projection
   c. Postvoiding emptied bladder, AP projection
   d. Retrograde cystogram, AP oblique projection (RPO position)

10. Fig. 18-25

   a. Excretory cystogram, AP projection
   b. Retrograde cystogram, AP projection
   c. Postvoiding emptied bladder, AP projection
   d. Retrograde cystogram, AP oblique projection (RPO position)

Fig. 18-23 Urinary examination radiograph.

Fig. 18-25 Urinary examination radiograph.

Self-Test: Anatomy and Positioning of the Urinary System

Instructions: Answer the following questions by selecting the best choice.

1. Which renal structure filters the blood?

   a. Glomerulus
   b. Major calyx
   c. Afferent arteriole
   d. Efferent arteriole

2. Which urinary excretory duct conveys urine from the bladder to outside the body?

   a. Ureter
   b. Urethra
   c. Afferent arteriole
   d. Efferent arteriole

3. Which body organ filters blood and produces urine as a by-product of waste material?

   a. Liver
   b. Spleen
   c. Kidney
   d. Pancreas

4. At which vertebral level is the superior border of the kidneys usually found?

   a. T10
   b. T12
   c. L2
   d. L4

5. What is the name of the opening on the medial border of a kidney?

   a. Pole
   b. Base
   c. Apex
   d. Hilum

6. Which of the following is an excretory examination used to demonstrate the upper urinary tract?

   a. Cystourethrography
   b. Retrograde urography
   c. Intravenous urography
   d. Retrograde cystography

7. Which examination has the ability to produce a radiographic image demonstrating renal cortical tissue well saturated with contrast medium?

   a. Cystourethrography
   b. Retrograde urography
   c. Intravenous urography
   d. Retrograde cystography

8. Which projection best demonstrates the mobility of the kidneys?

   a. AP projection with the patient supine
   b. AP projection with the patient upright
   c. Lateral projection with the patient lateral recumbent
   d. Lateral projection with the patient supine (dorsal decubitus position)

9. In intravenous urography, what is the purpose of applying compression pads over the distal ends of both ureters?

   a. To demonstrate ureteral reflux
   b. To demonstrate the mobility of the kidneys
   c. To retard the flow of opacified urine into the bladder
   d. To retard the flow of opacified urine from the bladder

10. Which of the following is *not* a reason for obtaining a scout radiograph with the patient recumbent for excretory urography?

    a. To evaluate exposure factors
    b. To demonstrate urinary calculi
    c. To determine the location of the kidneys
    d. To demonstrate the mobility of the kidneys

11. For excretory urography, what should an adult patient do just before getting on the examination table?

    a. Empty the bladder.
    b. Remove all jewelry.
    c. Drink 12 ounces of cold water.
    d. Drink 12 ounces of carbonated beverage.

12. What is the purpose of obtaining an AP projection radiograph of the kidneys 30 seconds after the bolus injection of a contrast medium in excretory urography?

    a. To demonstrate ureteral reflux
    b. To demonstrate opacified renal cortex
    c. To demonstrate opacified renal arteries
    d. To demonstrate the mobility of the kidneys

13. What is the purpose of tilting the patient and table 15 to 20 degrees Trendelenburg for the AP projection during excretory urography?

    a. To demonstrate distal ureters
    b. To demonstrate opacified renal cortex
    c. To demonstrate the base of the bladder
    d. To demonstrate the mobility of the kidneys

14. How many degrees should the patient be rotated for posterior (AP) oblique projections during excretory urography?

    a. 15
    b. 30
    c. 45
    d. 60

15. For intravenous urography of a child, what should the patient be given when the scout radiograph shows an excessive amount of intestinal gas overlying the kidneys?

    a. A laxative
    b. A cleansing enema
    c. 12 ounces of iced water
    d. 12 ounces of carbonated beverage

16. Which examination requires that the patient be placed on a special urographic-radiographic examination table?

    a. Cystourethrography
    b. Retrograde urography
    c. Intravenous urography
    d. Retrograde cystography

17. Which renal structures are not demonstrated during retrograde urographic examinations?

    a. Ureters
    b. Nephrons
    c. Minor calyces
    d. Major calyces

18. In addition to the AP projection, which projection would most likely be included in the radiographs for retrograde urography?

    a. PA projection
    b. PA oblique projection
    c. AP oblique projection
    d. AP projection, lateral decubitus position

19. What is the purpose of tilting the table 10 to 15 degrees Trendelenburg for retrograde urography?

    a. To demonstrate the ureters
    b. To demonstrate the mobility of the kidneys
    c. To produce a nephrogram effect in the kidneys
    d. To prevent contrast medium from escaping the kidneys

20. What is the purpose of raising the head of the table 35 to 40 degrees for retrograde urography?

    a. To demonstrate the ureters
    b. To position the patient for catheterization
    c. To produce a nephrogram effect in the kidneys
    d. To prevent contrast medium from escaping the kidneys

21. Which condition would most likely be demonstrated during voiding cystography?

    a. Renal cyst
    b. Renal calculi
    c. Ureteral reflux
    d. Hydronephrosis

22. For the AP axial projection of the bladder, how many degrees and in which direction should the central ray be directed?

    a. 15 degrees caudad
    b. 15 degrees cephalad
    c. 25 degrees caudad
    d. 25 degrees cephalad

23. For retrograde cystography, which projection should be performed to demonstrate the anterior and posterior walls of the bladder?

    a. Upright AP projection
    b. Recumbent AP projection
    c. Direct lateral projection
    d. AP projection, lateral decubitus position

24. For cystourethrography with an adult male patient, to which level of the patient should the cassette be centered?

    a. T12 vertebra
    b. L3 vertebra
    c. L5 vertebra
    d. Pubic symphysis

25. For cystourethrography with an adult male patient, which of the following should be used to obtain a radiograph while the patient is urinating?

    a. Recumbent PA projection
    b. Dorsal decubitus position
    c. Lateral decubitus position
    d. Recumbent AP oblique projection

 If your school has access to Mosby's Radiographic Instructional Series on Anatomy, Positioning, and Procedures, review Unit 18 at this time. Your instructor may request that you respond to the series' exercises on paper. This unit covers the following essential projections:

Urinary system
 AP projection
 AP oblique projection, RPO and LPO
 Lateral projection, right or left
 Lateral projection, dorsal decubitus
Pelvicalyceal system and ureters
 Retrograde urography
Urinary bladder
 AP and PA projections
 AP oblique projection, RPO or LPO
 Lateral projection, right or left
Male cystourethrography
 AP oblique projection, RPO or LPO

CHAPTER 19

Reproductive System

SECTION 1

Anatomy of the Reproductive System

Exercise 1

Instructions: This exercise pertains to the anatomy of the female reproductive system. Identify structures, fill in missing words, provide a short answer, or match columns for each item.

1. Identify each lettered structure shown in Fig. 19-1.

   A. _____

   B. _____

   C. _____

   D. _____

   E. _____

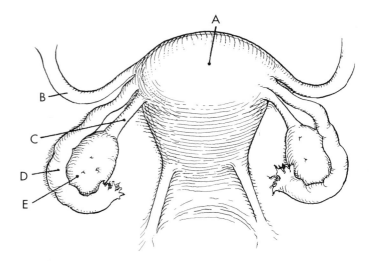

Fig. 19-1 Superoposterior view of the uterus, ovaries, and uterine tubes.

2. Identify each lettered structure shown in Fig. 19-2.

A. _____

B. _____

C. _____

D. _____

E. _____

F. _____

G. _____

H. _____

I. _____

J. _____

K. _____

L. _____

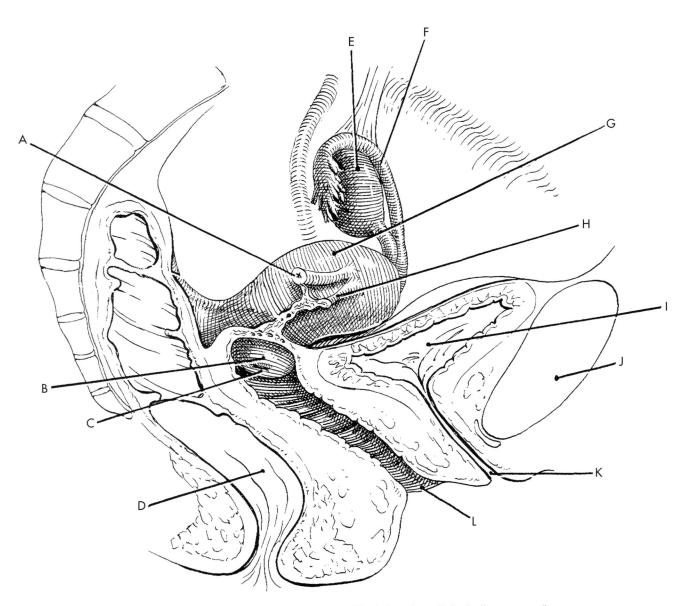

Fig. 19-2 Sagittal section showing the relation of the internal genitalia to the surrounding structures.

3. The female gonads are called the

   _____.

4. Female reproductive cells are called

   _____.

5. The structure that conveys an ovum from a gonad to the

   uterus is the _____ tube.

6. The number of uterine tubes in the typical adult female is

   _____.

7. The pear-shaped muscular organ of the female reproduc-

   tive system is the _____.

8. Name the four main parts of the uterus.

9. What part of the uterus is referred to as the neck?

   _____

10. Match the uterine structures in Column A with the defini-
    tions in Column B.

   Column A   **Column B**

   _____ 1. Body   a. Superiormost portion

   _____ 2. Fundus   b. Cylindrical vaginal end

   _____ 3. Cervix   c. Mucosal lining of the uter-
                                  ine cavity
   _____ 4. Isthmus
                               d. Constricted area adjacent to
   _____ 5. Endometrium   the vaginal end

                               e. Where ligaments attach the
                                  uterus within the pelvis

Exercise 2

Instructions: This exercise pertains to the anatomy of the male reproductive system. Identify structures or fill in missing words for each item.

1. Identify each lettered structure shown in Fig.19-3.

   A. _____

   B. _____

   C. _____

   D. _____

   E. _____

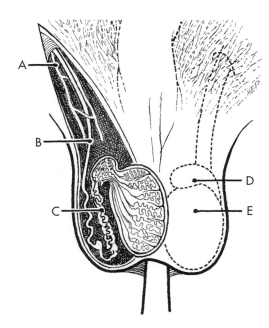

Fig. 19-3 Frontal section of the testes and ductus deferens.

2. Identify each lettered structure in Fig. 19-4.

A. _____

B. _____

C. _____

D. _____

E. _____

F. _____

G. _____

3. Identify each lettered structure shown in Fig. 19-5.

A. _____

B. _____

C. _____

D. _____

E. _____

F. _____

G. _____

H. _____

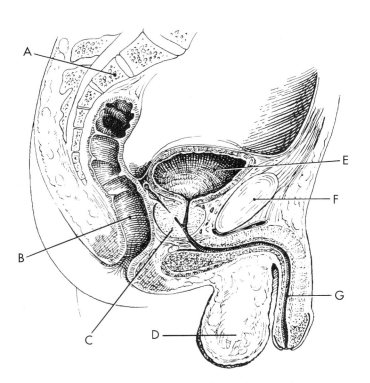

Fig. 19-4 Sagittal section showing the male genital system.

Fig. 19-5 Sagittal section through the male pelvis.

4. The male gonads are called the

   _____.

5. Male reproductive cells are called

   _____.

6. The oblong structure attached to each testicle is the

   _____.

7. The excretory channel that allows male germ cells to pass from a gonad to the urethra is the

   _____ _____.

8. The union of the ductus deferens and the seminal vesicle duct forms the _____ duct.

9. The accessory genital organ that is composed of muscular and glandular tissues is the _____.

10. The ducts from the prostate open into the proximal portion of the _____.

SECTION 2

Radiography of the Reproductive System

Exercise 1: Radiography of the Female Reproductive System

Instructions: Although other imaging modalities have reduced the demand for radiographic examinations of the female reproductive system, some facilities still radiographically demonstrate female reproductive structures. This exercise pertains to radiographic visualization of the female reproductive system. Match columns of relevant information or select the correct answer from a list for each item.

1. Match each radiographic examination from Column A with the type of patient from Column B who is most likely to undergo that type of examination.

   Column A

   ____ 1. Fetography

   ____ 2. Pelvimetry

   ____ 3. Vaginography

   ____ 4. Placentography

   ____ 5. Pelvic pneumography

   ____ 6. Hysterosalpingography

   Column B

   a. Pregnant patient

   b. Nongravid patient

2. Match the descriptions in Column A with the corresponding type of examination in Column B. Some descriptions may have more than one examination associated with them. Examinations will be used more than once.

Column A

_____ 1. Determines pelvic diameters

_____ 2. Uses a Colcher-Sussman ruler

_____ 3. Helps determine placenta previa

_____ 4. Requires a gaseous contrast agent

_____ 5. Requires the use of a contrast agent

_____ 6. Requires a radiopaque contrast agent

_____ 7. Investigates the patency of uterine tubes

_____ 8. Largely replaced by diagnostic ultrasound

_____ 9. Performed to demonstrate a fetus in utero

_____ 10. Introduces a contrast agent into the vaginal canal

_____ 11. Introduces a contrast agent through a uterine cannula

_____ 12. Introduces a contrast agent directly into the peritoneal cavity

_____ 13. Should be performed about 10 days after the onset of menstruation

_____ 14. Performed to determine the size, shape, and position of the uterus and uterine tubes

_____ 15. Performed to demonstrate congenital abnormalities of the muscular structure that extends from the cervix to the external genitalia

Column B

a. Fetography

b. Pelvimetry

c. Vaginography

d. Placentography

e. Pelvic pneumography

f. Hysterosalpingography

3. Figs. 19-6 through 19-10 are representative examinations of the female reproductive system. Examine the images, then select the best answer from the list provided for each image.

i. Fig. 19-6:
   a. Pelvimetry
   b. Vaginography
   c. Pelvic pneumography
   d. Hysterosalpingography

Uterine tube

Normal contrast "spill" into peritoneal cavity

Body of uterus

Speculum

Fig. 19-6 Radiograph of the female reproductive system.

ii. Fig. 19-7:
   a. Fetography
   b. Vaginography
   c. Pelvic pneumography
   d. Hysterosalpingography

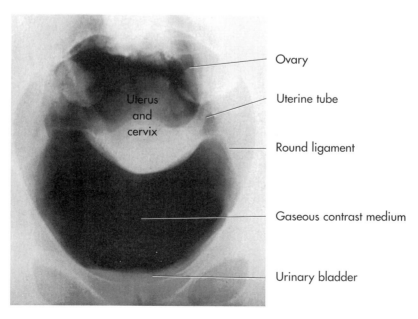

Ovary

Uterus and cervix

Uterine tube

Round ligament

Gaseous contrast medium

Urinary bladder

Fig. 19-7 Radiograph of the female reproductive system.

iii. Fig. 19-8:

    a. Pelvimetry

    b. Vaginography

    c. Pelvic pneumography

    d. Hysterosalpingography

iv. Fig. 19-9:

    a. Pelvimetry

    b. Fetography

    c. Placentography

    d. Hysterosalpingography

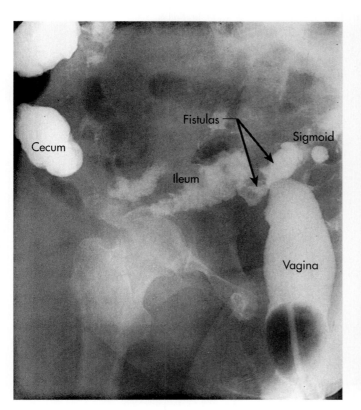

Fig. 19-8 Radiograph of the female reproductive system.

Fig. 19-9 Radiograph of the female reproductive system.

v. Fig. 19-10:

    a. Pelvimetry
    b. Fetography
    c. Placentography
    d. Pelvic pneumography

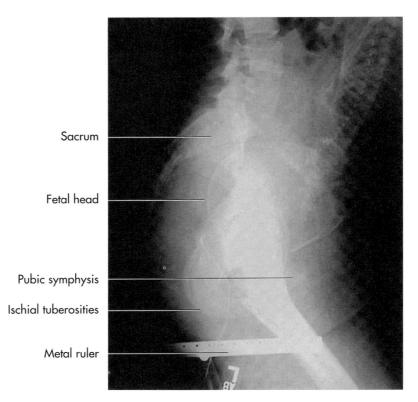

Sacrum

Fetal head

Pubic symphysis

Ischial tuberosities

Metal ruler

Fig. 19-10 Radiograph of the female reproductive system.

Exercise 2: Radiography of the Male Reproductive System

Instructions: Although the demand for radiographic visualization of the male reproductive system has greatly decreased in recent years because of advances with diagnostic ultrasound, some facilities still radiographically demonstrate male reproductive structures. This exercise pertains to radiographic visualization of the male reproductive system. Provide a short answer for each question.

1. What type of contrast medium is used for radiographic examination of the seminal ducts?

_____

2. Why might a radiolucent contrast medium be injected into the scrotum for epididymography?

3. What accessory organ of the male reproductive system can be radiographically examined?

_____

4. What body position is preferred for radiography of the prostate? Explain why.

5. For PA projections of the prostate, how many degrees and in which direction should the central ray be directed?

_____

Self-Test: Reproductive System

Instructions: Answer the following questions by selecting the best choice.

1. Which structures are part of the female reproductive system?
   a. Ovaries, uterus, and fallopian tubes
   b. Ovaries, testes, and ductus deferens
   c. Epididymis, uterus, and fallopian tubes
   d. Epididymis, testes, and ductus deferens

2. Which part of the uterus is most superior?
   a. Body
   b. Cervix
   c. Fundus
   d. Isthmus

3. Which structure conveys female reproductive cells from a gonad to the uterus?
   a. Urethra
   b. Uterine tube
   c. Ductus deferens
   d. Ejaculatory duct

4. Which structure produces female reproductive cells?
   a. Ovary
   b. Uterus
   c. Testicle
   d. Epididymis

5. Which structure produces spermatozoa?
   a. Ovary
   b. Testicle
   c. Prostate
   d. Epididymis

6. Which structure conveys male reproductive cells from a gonad to the urethra?
   a. Uterine tube
   b. Fallopian tube
   c. Ductus deferens
   d. Ejaculatory duct

7. Which structure is attached to each male gonad?
   a. Urethra
   b. Prostate
   c. Epididymis
   d. Ejaculatory duct

8. Which examination can be performed on a pregnant patient?
   a. Fetography
   b. Prostatography
   c. Pelvic pneumography
   d. Hysterosalpingography

9. Which examination can be performed on a nongravid patient?
   a. Fetography
   b. Pelvimetry
   c. Placentography
   d. Hysterosalpingography

10. Which examination introduces contrast medium through a uterine cannula?
    a. Fetography
    b. Pelvimetry
    c. Vaginography
    d. Hysterosalpingography

11. Which examination is performed to verify the patency of uterine tubes?
    a. Fetography
    b. Pelvimetry
    c. Placentography
    d. Hysterosalpingography

12. Which examination determines pelvic diameters?
    a. Fetography
    b. Pelvimetry
    c. Placentography
    d. Hysterosalpingography

13. Which type of contrast medium is preferred for hysterosalpingography?
    a. Oily viscous
    b. Water-soluble
    c. Barium sulfate

14. When should a hysterosalpingographic examination be performed?
    a. After the first trimester
    b. During the first trimester
    c. 10 days after the onset of menstruation
    d. 10 days before the onset of menstruation

15. Which projection is preferred for prostatography?
    a. AP axial
    b. PA axial
    c. Lateral
    d. AP oblique (RPO position)

If your school has access to Mosby's Radiographic Instructional Series on Anatomy, Positioning, and Procedures, review Unit 19 at this time. Your instructor may request that you respond to the series' exercises on paper. This unit covers the following examinations:

Female radiography
Nongravid patient
Gravid patient
Fetography
Radiographic pelvimetry and cephalometry
Pelvimetry
Localization of intrauterine devices
Male radiography
Seminal ducts
Prostate

CHAPTER 20

Skull

SECTION 1

Osteology of the Skull

Exercise 1

Instructions: This exercise pertains to the osteology of the skull. Identify structures for each illustration.

1. Identify each lettered structure shown in Fig. 20-1.

A. _____

B. _____

C. _____

D. _____

E. _____

F. _____

G. _____

H. _____

I. _____

J. _____

K. _____

L. _____

M. _____

N. _____

O. _____

P. _____

Q. _____

R. _____

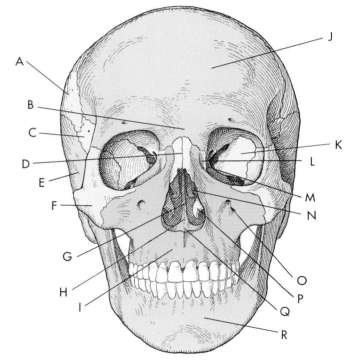

Fig. 20-1 Anterior aspect of the skull.

2. Identify each lettered structure shown in Fig. 20-2.

A. _____

B. _____

C. _____

D. _____

E. _____

F. _____

G. _____

H. _____

I. _____

J. _____

K. _____

L. _____

M. _____ (fontanel)

N. _____ (suture)

O. _____

P. _____ (suture)

Q. _____ (fontanel)

R. _____ (suture)

S. _____

T. _____

U. _____

V. _____

W. _____

X. _____

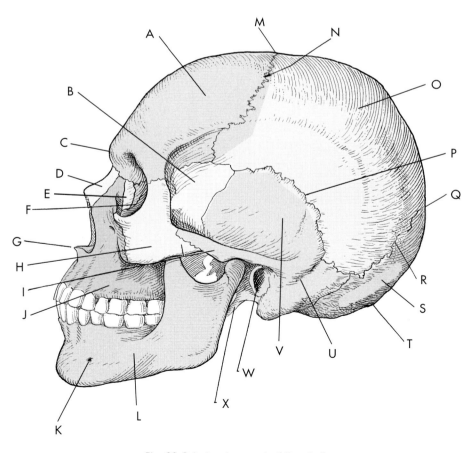

Fig. 20-2 Lateral aspect of the skull.

3. Identify each lettered structure shown in Fig. 20-3.

A. _____   L. _____

B. _____   M. _____

C. _____   N. _____

D. _____   O. _____

E. _____   P. _____

F. _____   Q. _____

G. _____   R. _____

H. _____   S. _____

I. _____   T. _____

J. _____   U. _____

K. _____   V. _____

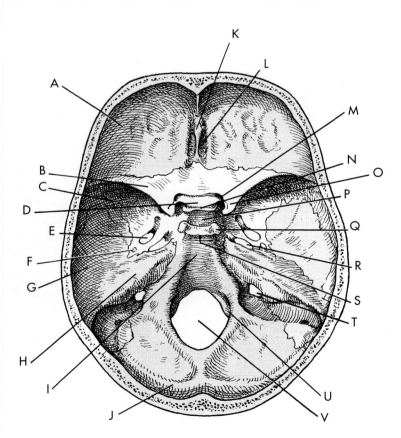

Fig. 20-3 Superior aspect of the cranial base.

4. Identify each lettered structure shown in Fig. 20-4.

A. _____

B. _____

C. _____

D. _____

E. _____

F. _____

G. _____

H. _____

I. _____

J. _____

K. _____

L. _____

M. _____

N. _____

O. _____

P. _____

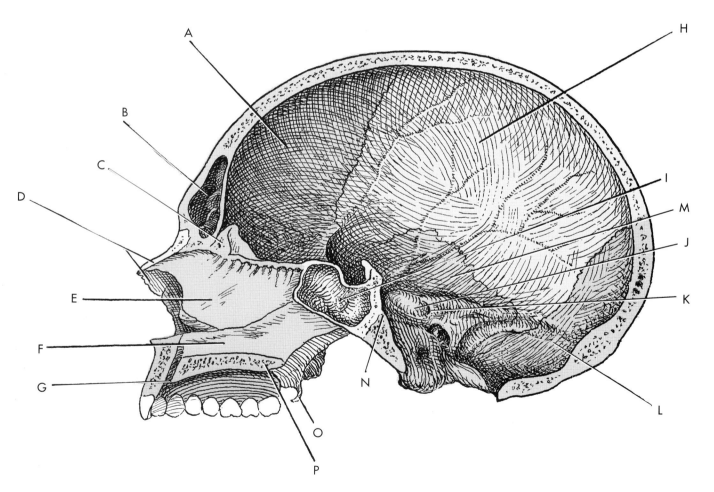

Fig. 20-4 Lateral aspect of the interior of the cranium.

5. Identify each lettered structure shown in Fig. 20-5.

A. _____

B. _____

C. _____

D. _____

E. _____

F. _____

G. _____

6. Identify each lettered structure shown in Fig. 20-6.

A. _____

B. _____

C. _____

D. _____

E. _____

F. _____

G. _____

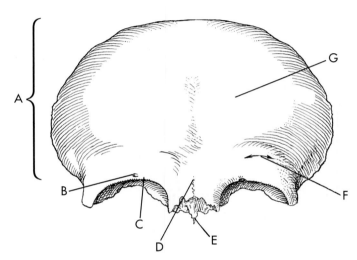

Fig. 20-5 Anterior aspect of the frontal bone.

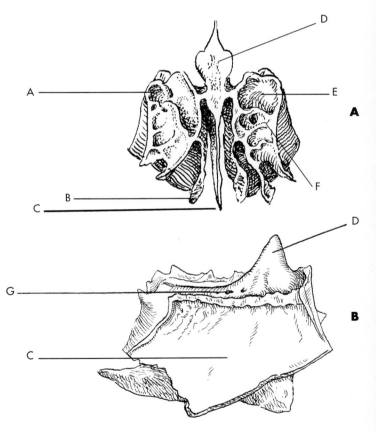

Fig. 20-6 Two illustrations of the ethmoid bone: **A,** the anterior aspect; **B,** the lateral aspect with the labyrinth removed.

7. Identify the four angles and the four articulating borders of the left parietal bone shown in Fig. 20-7.

A. Articulates with the_____ bone

B. _____ angle

C. Articulates with the_____ bone

D. _____ angle

E. _____ angle

F. Articulates with the_____ bone

G. _____ angle

H. Articulates with the_____ bone

8. Identify each lettered structure shown in Fig. 20-8.

A. _____

B. _____

C. _____

D. _____

E. _____

F. _____

G. _____

H. _____

I. _____

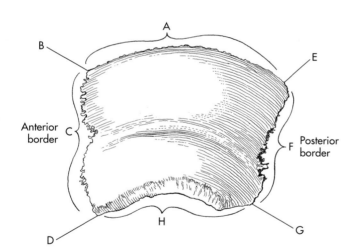

Fig. 20-7 External surface of the left parietal bone.

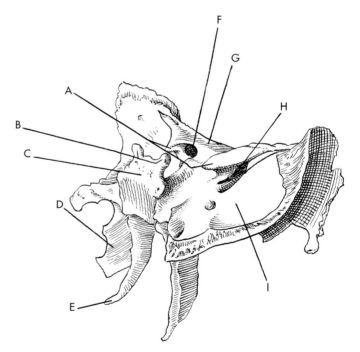

Fig. 20-8 Oblique view of the upper and lateroposterior aspects of the sphenoid bone.

9. Identify each lettered structure shown in Fig. 20-9.

A. _____ D. _____

B. _____ E. _____

C. _____

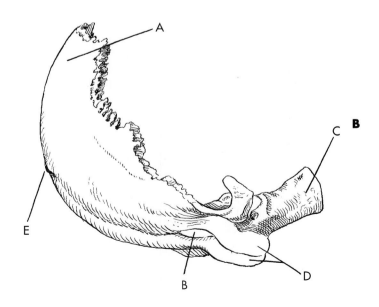

Fig. 20-9 Two illustrations of the occipital bone: **A,** the external surface; **B,** the lateroinferior surface.

10. Identify each lettered structure shown in Fig. 20-10.

A. _____   F. _____

B. _____   G. _____

C. _____   H. _____

D. _____   I. _____

E. _____

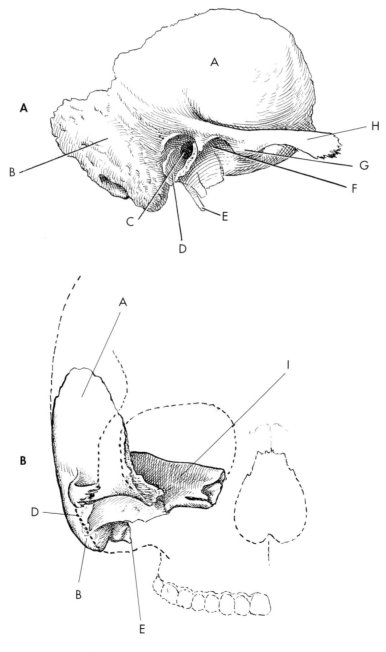

Fig. 20-10 Two illustrations of the temporal bone: **A,** the lateral aspect; **B,** the anterior aspect in relation to the surrounding structures.

11. Identify each lettered structure shown in Fig. 20-11.

A. _____   H. _____

B. _____   I. _____

C. _____   J. _____

D. _____   K. _____

E. _____   L. _____

F. _____   M. _____

G. _____   N. _____

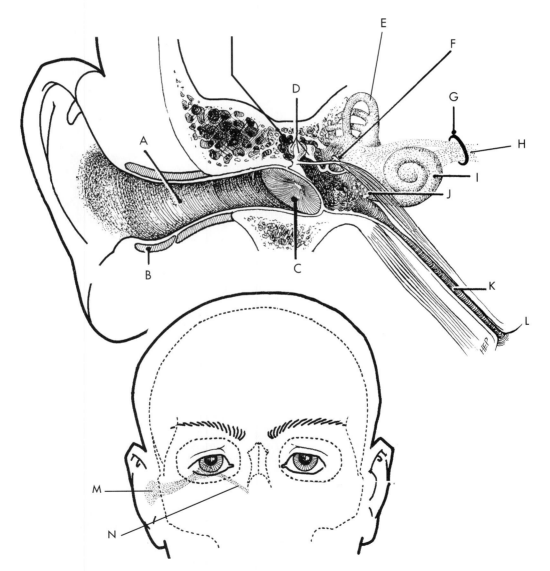

Fig. 20-11 Frontal section through the right ear showing the internal structures.

12. Identify each lettered structure shown in Fig. 20-12.

A. _____

B. _____

C. _____

D. _____

E. _____

F. _____

G. _____

H. _____

I. _____

J. _____

K. _____

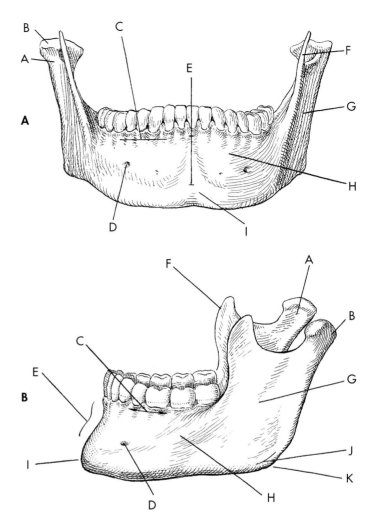

Fig. 20-12 Two illustrations of the mandible: **A,** the anterior aspect; **B,** the lateral aspect.

13. Identify each lettered structure shown in Fig. 20-13.

A. _____

B. _____

C. _____

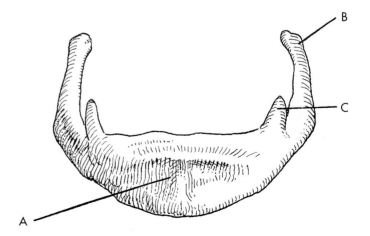

Fig. 20-13 Anterior aspect of the hyoid.

Exercise 2

Instructions: Use the following clues to complete the cross-word puzzle below. All answers refer to the skull.

ACROSS

1. Perpendicular _____
4. Midpoint of the frontonasal suture
5. This bone has wings
7. Vertical part of the frontal bone
8. _____ galli
9. Number of cranial bones
12. Densest part of the cranial floor
13. Articulates frontal bone with parietals
16. Fibrous cranial joint
19. Anterior fontanel
20. Posterior fontanel
21. Forms top of the cranium
22. Posterior part of the skull
23. Eyebrow arches

DOWN

1. Inferior sphenoidal process
2. Sphenoidal endocrine
3. _____ turcica
5. Lateral suture
6. Long and narrow skull
10. Average skull
11. Smooth frontal elevation
14. Posterior to the nasal bones
15. Ear bone
17. Where occipital bone joins parietals
18. Forehead bone
19. Anteroinferior occipital part

Exercise 3

Instructions: Match the structures (Column A) with the cranial bones on which they are found (Column B).

Column A	Column B
____ 1. Nasion	a. Frontal
____ 2. Glabella	b. Ethmoid
____ 3. Four angles	c. Parietal
____ 4. Lesser wing	d. Sphenoid
____ 5. Greater wing	e. Temporal
____ 6. Two condyles	f. Occipital
____ 7. Crista galli	
____ 8. Sella turcica	
____ 9. Foramen magnum	
____ 10. Cribriform plate	
____ 11. Mastoid process	
____ 12. Basilar portion	
____ 13. Petrous portion	
____ 14. Pterygoid hamulus	
____ 15. Zygomatic process	
____ 16. Supraorbital margin	
____ 17. Perpendicular plate	
____ 18. Lateral pterygoid process	
____ 19. Anterior clinoid processes	
____ 20. Posterior clinoid processes	

Exercise 4

Instructions: Match the statements (Column A) with the facial bone terms to which they refer (Column B). Only one selection from Column B applies to each statement in Column A. Not all terms from Column B should be used.

Column A	Column B
____ 1. Cheek bone	a. Head
____ 2. Largest facial bone	b. Body
____ 3. Number of facial bones	c. Nasal
____ 4. Forms bridge of the nose	d. Hyoid
____ 5. Vertical mandibular portion	e. Ramus
____ 6. Found in the roof of the mouth	f. Vomer
____ 7. Midpoint of the anterior nasal spine	g. Gonion
____ 8. Articulating process of the mandible	h. Twelve
____ 9. Spongy processes that hold the teeth	i. Fourteen
____ 10. Anterior part of the mandibular ramus	j. Lacrimal
____ 11. Landmark at the angle of the mandible	k. Alveolar
____ 12. Found in the medial walls of the orbits	l. Condyle
____ 13. Forms the inferior portion of the nasal septum	m. Zygoma
____ 14. Horseshoe-shaped mandibular portion	n. Palatine
____ 15. Thin, scroll-like bones that extend horizontally inside nasal cavity	o. Maxillae
	p. Coronoid
	q. Mandible
	r. Acanthion
	s. Inferior conchae
	t. Mental protuberance

Exercise 5

Instructions: This exercise is a comprehensive review of the osteology and arthrology of the skull. Fill in missing words or provide a short answer for each item.

1. The bones of the skull are divided into two major groups,

   the _____ bones and the

   _____ bones.

2. List by name and quantity the cranial bones.

3. List by name and quantity the facial bones.

4. The bones of the cranial vault are classified as

   _____ bones.

5. The inner layer of spongy tissue found inside cranial bones

   is called _____.

6. The two fontanels located on the midsagittal plane of the

   skull are the _____ and the

   _____.

7. The fontanel located at the junction of the coronal and

   sagittal sutures is the _____.

8. The fontanel located at the junction of the lambdoidal and

   sagittal sutures is the _____.

9. List the three classifications of fundamental skull shapes and indicate the number of degrees of angulation (formed by the petrous pyramids and the midsagittal plane) for each classification.

10. The bone that forms the anterior portion of the cranium is

    the _____ bone.

11. The cranial bone located between the orbits and posterior

    to the nasal bones is the _____ bone.

12. The cranial bones that form the vertex and most of the

    sides of the cranium are the _____
    bones.

13. The prominent bulge of a parietal bone is called the pari-

    etal _____.

14. The two parietal bones join together to form the

    _____ suture.

15. The two parietal bones articulate with the frontal bone to

    form the _____ suture.

16. The two parietal bones articulate posteriorly with the

    _____ bone.

17. The two parietal bones and the occipital bone join together

    to form the _____ suture.

18. The cranial bone that provides a depression to house the

    pituitary gland is the _____ bone.

19. The cranial bone that forms the posteroinferior portion of

    the cranium is the _____ bone.

20. The portion of the occipital bone that projects anteriorly from the foramen magnum is the

_____ portion.

21. The large opening of the occipital bone through which part of the medulla oblongata passes is the

_____ _____.

22. The basilar portion of the occipital bone fuses anteriorly

with the body of the _____ bone.

23. The structure that articulates with the occipital condyles is

the _____.

24. The middle portion of the cranial base is formed by the

_____ bone.

25. The organs of hearing are located in the

_____ bone.

26. The structure that separates the external acoustic meatus from the auditory ossicles is the

_____ membrane.

27. The process of the temporal bone that encloses radiographically significant air cells is the

_____ process.

28. The thickest and densest portion of bone in the cranium is

the _____

_____.

29. The petrous portion is a part of the

_____ bone.

30. The fibrocartilaginous, oval-shaped portion of the external

ear is the _____.

31. The three auditory ossicles are the

_____, _____,

and the _____.

32. The zygomatic process projects anteriorly from the

_____ bone.

33. The bone that forms part of the cranial base between the greater wings of the sphenoid bone and the occipital bone

is the _____ bone.

34. The facial bones that form the bridge of the nose are the

_____ bones.

35. The anterior portion of the medial walls of the orbits is

formed by the _____ bones.

36. The largest of the immovable bones of the face is the

_____ bone.

37. The body of each maxilla contains a large, pyramidal

cavity called the _____

_____.

38. The thick ridge on the inferior border of the maxillary bone

that supports the teeth is the _____

_____.

39. The anterior nasal spine projects superiorly from the

_____.

40. The radiographically significant landmark that is the midpoint of the anterior nasal spine is the

_____.

41. The facial bones that form the inferolateral portion of the

orbital margin are the _____ bones.

42. The facial bones that form the prominence of the cheeks

are the _____ bones.

43. The facial bones that form the posterior one fourth of the

roof of the mouth are the _____ bones.

44. The scroll-like bony tissues that extend along the lateral walls of the nasal cavity are the

    _____ _____

    _____.

45. The facial bone forming the inferior part of the nasal septum is the _____.

46. The largest and densest bone of the face is the

    _____.

47. The portion of the mandible that extends superiorly from the posterior aspect of the mandibular body is the

    _____.

48. The U-shaped bone located at the base of the tongue is the

    _____ bone.

49. The two processes that extend superiorly from a mandibular ramus are the _____ and the

    _____ process.

50. The part of the mandible that articulates with the mandibular fossa of the temporal bone to form the temporomandibular joint is the _____.

SECTION 2

Radiography of the Skull

Exercise 1: Skull Topography

Instructions: This exercise pertains to positioning landmarks used in skull radiography. Identify landmarks or provide a short answer for each item.

1. Identify each lettered positioning landmark shown in Fig. 20-14.

A. _____

B. _____

C. _____

D. _____

E. _____

F. _____

G. _____

H. _____

I. _____

J. _____

2. Identify each lettered positioning landmark shown in Fig. 20-15.

A. _____

B. _____

C. _____

D. _____

E. _____

F. _____

G. _____

H. _____

I. _____

J. _____

K. _____

Fig. 20-15 Lateral aspect landmarks.

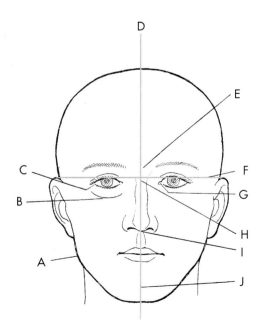

Fig. 20-14 Anterior aspect landmarks.

3. Match the definitions in Column A with the appropriate term from Column B. Each term may be used only once.

Column A

_____ 1. Midpoint of the fronto-nasal suture

_____ 2. Midpoint of the anterior nasal spine

_____ 3. Posterior surface of the occipital bone

_____ 4. Smooth elevation between the superciliary arches

_____ 5. Lateral aspect of each orbit; where the two eyelids originate

_____ 6. Angle of the mandible; lateroposterior aspect of the mandible

_____ 7. Superior aspect of the cranium; where the parietal bones join together

_____ 8. Raised prominence just above each orbit on the frontal bone; coincides with the eyebrows

_____ 9. Midpoint of the mental protuberance; anterior aspect of the mandible; where the two mandibular bodies join together

Column B

a. Inion

b. Vertex

c. Nasion

d. Gonion

e. Glabella

f. Acanthion

g. Mental point

h. Outer canthus

i. Superciliary arch

4. Match the definitions in Column A with the appropriate terms in Column B. The terms represent skull topography lines or planes. Each term may be used once, more than once, or not at all.

Column A

_____ 1. Line extending across the front through both eyes

_____ 2. Plane dividing the skull into equal right and left halves

_____ 3. Line extending from the glabella to the anterior aspect of the maxilla

_____ 4. Line extending from the external acoustic meatus to the outer canthus

_____ 5. Line extending from the external acoustic meatus to the inferior margin of the orbit

_____ 6. Line extending from the external acoustic meatus to the midpoint of the anterior nasal spine

_____ 7. Line extending from the external acoustic meatus to the smooth elevation between the superciliary arches

Column B

a. Sagittal

b. Midsagittal

c. Midcoronal

d. Orbitomeatal

e. Interpupillary

f. Glabellomeatal

g. Acanthiomeatal

h. Glabelloalveolar

i. Infraorbitomeatal

5. How many degrees exist in the angles formed by the following lines?

a. Orbitomeatal and infraorbitomeatal lines: _____

b. Orbitomeatal and glabellomeatal lines: _____

Exercise 2: Positioning for the Cranium

Instructions: The typical radiographic evaluation of the skull, usually referred to as a skull series, involves a series of radiographs that may include a PA or AP projection, an AP axial projection, a full basal view, and one or two lateral views. This exercise pertains to those projections. Identify structures, fill in missing words, provide a short answer, select from a list, or choose true or false (explaining any statement you believe to be false) for each item.

Items 1 through 12 pertain to the *lateral projection.* Examine Fig. 20-16 as you answer the following items.

Fig. 20-16 Lateral skull.

1. Which size cassette should be used for average-sized adult skulls, and how should it be placed in the cassette holder?
   a. 18 × 24 cm; crosswise
   b. 18 × 24 cm; lengthwise
   c. 24 × 30 cm; crosswise
   d. 24 × 30 cm; lengthwise

2. Indicate how the midsagittal plane and the interpupillary line should be positioned—perpendicular or parallel—with reference to the plane of the cassette.

   a. Midsagittal plane: _____

   b. Interpupillary line: _____

3. Which positioning line of the head should be parallel with the plane of the cassette?
   a. Interpupillary line
   b. Glabelloalveolar line
   c. Infraorbitomeatal line

4. Which structure should be nearest to the center of the midline of the grid?
   a. Acanthion
   b. Zygoma bone
   c. Outer canthus
   d. External acoustic meatus

5. To what level of the patient should the cassette be centered?

6. Describe how and to where the central ray should be directed.

7. For cross-table lateral projections with the patient supine, which procedure should be performed to ensure that the entire cranium is included in the image?
   a. Elevate the head on a radiolucent sponge.
   b. Increase the source-to-image receptor distance (SID) to 72 inches.
   c. Use an 18- × 24-cm image receptor positioned lengthwise relative to the skull.

8. True or False. For cross-table lateral projections with the patient supine, the central ray should enter the side of the head at a point 2 inches (5 cm) anterior to the external acoustic meatus.

9. True or False. For cross-table lateral projections with the patient supine, a vertically-oriented grid cassette should be placed against the side of interest.

10. From the list below, circle the eight evaluation criteria that indicate the patient was properly positioned for a lateral projection.

    a. The petrous ridges should be symmetric.
    b. The sella turcica should be seen in profile.
    c. The orbital roofs should be superimposed.
    d. The mastoid regions should be superimposed.
    e. The mandible should not overlap the cervical vertebrae.
    f. The greater wings of sphenoid should be superimposed.
    g. The temporomandibular joints should be superimposed.
    h. The external acoustic meatuses should be superimposed.
    i. The dorsum sellae should be within the foramen magnum.
    j. The entire cranium should be demonstrated without rotation or tilt.
    k. The mental protuberance should be superimposed over the anterior frontal bone.
    l. The distance from the lateral border of the skull to the lateral border of the orbit should be equal on both sides.

11. Fig. 20-17 shows two diagrams of a recumbent patient with the midsagittal plane improperly aligned. Examine the diagrams and explain how the position of the patient in each should be adjusted to properly align the midsagittal plane with the cassette.

    a. Diagram *A*:

    _____

    _____

    _____

    b. Diagram *B*:

    _____

    _____

    _____

Asthenic or hyposthenic patient

Hypersthenic patient

Fig. 20-17 Adjusting the midsagittal plane with the patient in the recumbent position: **A,** asthenic or hyposthenic patient; **B,** hypersthenic patient.

12. Identify each lettered structure shown in Fig. 20-18.

A. _____

B. _____

C. _____

D. _____

E. _____

F. _____

G. _____

Fig. 20-18 Lateral skull.

Items 13 through 20 pertain to *PA and PA axial projections.* Examine Figs. 20-19 and 20-20 as you answer the following items.

Fig. 20-19 PA skull.

Fig. 20-20 PA axial skull.

13. Indicate how the midsagittal plane and the orbitomeatal line should be positioned—perpendicular or parallel—with reference to the plane of the cassette.

a. Midsagittal plane: _____

b. Orbitomeatal line: _____

14. Which parts of the patient's facial area should be in contact with the table or vertical grid device?
   a. Chin and nose
   b. Chin and cheek
   c. Forehead and nose
   d. Forehead and cheek

15. To demonstrate each of the following structures (Column A), identify how the central ray should be directed (Column B) with the patient positioned for a PA projection of the skull.

Column A	Column B
____ 1. Frontal bone	a. Perpendicular
____ 1. General survey	b. 15 degrees caudad
____ 1. Rotundum foramina	c. 20 to 25 degrees caudad
____ 1. Superior orbital fissures	d. 25 to 30 degrees caudad

16. The central ray should exit the skull at the

_____.

17. The cassette should be centered to the skull at the level of

the _____.

18. What breathing instructions should be given to the patient?

_____

19. From the list below, circle the five evaluation criteria that indicate the patient was properly positioned for either PA or PA axial projections.

   a. The petrous ridges should be symmetric.
   b. The orbital roofs should be superimposed.
   c. The entire cranial perimeter should be included.
   d. The mandible should not overlap the cervical vertebrae.
   e. The dorsum sellae should be within the foramen magnum.
   f. The mental protuberance should be superimposed over the anterior frontal bone
   g. The frontal bone should be penetrated without excessive density at the lateral borders of the skull.
   h. The distance from the lateral border of the skull to the lateral border of the orbit should be equal on both sides.
   i. The petrous pyramids should lie in the lower one third of the orbit with a central ray angulation of 15 degrees caudad, and should fill the orbits with no central ray angulation.

20. Identify each lettered structure shown in Fig. 20-21.

   A. _____

   B. _____

   C. _____

   D. _____

   E. _____

   F. _____

   G. _____

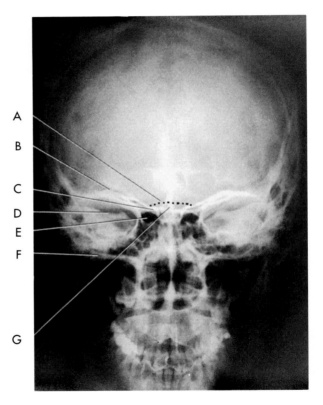

Fig. 20-21 PA skull.

Items 21 through 27 pertain to *AP and AP axial projections.* Examine Figs. 20-22 and 20-23 as you answer the following items.

Fig. 20-22 AP skull.

Fig. 20-23 AP axial skull.

21. Indicate how the midsagittal plane and the orbitomeatal line should be positioned—perpendicular or parallel—with reference to the plane of the cassette.

    a. Midsagittal plane: _____

    b. Orbitomeatal line: _____

22. For the AP projection, the central ray should be directed

    _____ (caudally, cephalically, or perpendicularly).

23. For the AP axial projection, the central ray should be

    directed _____ (caudally, cephalically, or perpendicularly).

24. When performing either the AP or AP axial projection for general surveys of the skull, to where on the skull should the central ray be directed?
    a. Nasion
    b. Acanthion
    c. Tip of the nose

25. Which of the following image characteristics indicates that a general survey image of the skull is an AP projection instead of a PA projection?
    a. The petrous ridges are symmetric.
    b. The petrous pyramids fill the orbits.
    c. The orbits are considerably magnified.
    d. The entire cranial perimeter is demonstrated.

26. From the list below, circle the five evaluation criteria that indicate the patient was properly positioned for either the AP or AP axial projections.
    a. The petrous ridges should be symmetric.
    b. The orbital roofs should be superimposed.
    c. The entire cranial perimeter should be included.
    d. The mandible should not overlap the cervical vertebrae.
    e. The dorsum sellae should be within the foramen magnum.
    f. The mental protuberance should be superimposed over the anterior frontal bone.
    g. The frontal bone should be penetrated without excessive density at the lateral borders of the skull.
    h. The distance from the lateral border of the skull to the lateral border of the orbit should be equal on both sides.
    i. The petrous pyramids should lie in the lower one third of the orbit, with a central ray angulation of 15 degrees caudad, and should fill the orbits with no central ray angulation.
    j. The petrous pyramids should lie in the lower one third of the orbit, with a central ray angulation of 15 degrees cephalically, and should fill the orbits with no central ray angulation.

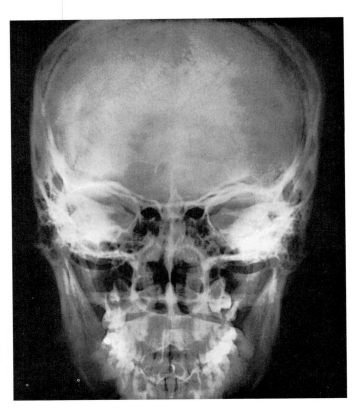

Fig. 20-24 Two views of the skull.

27. Fig. 20-24 shows two skull radiographs: one AP and one
AP axial. Examine each image and state how the central
ray was directed by indicating how specific structures appear in relation to the surrounding structures.

a. Diagram *A*:

_____

_____

_____

b. Diagram *B*:

_____

_____

_____

Items 28 through 35 pertain to the *AP axial projection (Towne method)*. Examine Fig. 20-25 as you answer the following items.

Fig. 20-25 AP axial skull (Towne method).

28. Which size cassette should be used for average-sized adult skulls, and how should it be placed in the cassette holder?
    a. 18 × 24 cm; crosswise
    b. 18 × 24 cm; lengthwise
    c. 24 × 30 cm; crosswise
    d. 24 × 30 cm; lengthwise

29. To what level of the patient should the upper border of the cassette be aligned?
    a. Nasion
    b. Glabella
    c. Highest point of the vertex

30. In addition to the midsagittal plane, either the

    _____ line or the

    _____ line must be perpendicular to the plane of the cassette.

31. Which two central ray angulations could be used to properly perform the AP axial projection?
    a. 30 degrees caudad and 37 degrees caudad
    b. 30 degrees caudad and 37 degrees cephalad
    c. 30 degrees cephalad and 37 degrees caudad
    d. 30 degrees cephalad and 37 degrees cephalad

32. Where exactly on the patient's head should the central ray enter?
    a. 1 inch (2.5 cm) above the nasion
    b. 1 inch (2.5 cm) below the nasion
    c. 2 to 2½ inches (5 to 6.25 cm) above the glabella
    d. 2 to 2½ inches (5 to 6.25 cm) below the glabella

33. What positioning characteristic determines the number of degrees that the central ray should be angled?

34. From the list below, circle the four evaluation criteria that indicate the patient was properly positioned for the AP axial projection, Towne method.
    a. The orbital roofs should be superimposed.
    b. The petrous pyramids should be symmetric.
    c. The mandible should not overlap the cervical vertebrae.
    d. The petrous pyramids should lie in the lower one third of the orbits.
    e. The mental protuberance should be superimposed over the anterior frontal bone.
    f. The occipital bone should be penetrated without excessive density at the lateral borders of the skull.
    g. The dorsum sellae and posterior clinoid processes should be visualized within the foramen magnum.
    h. The distance from the lateral border of the skull to the lateral border of the orbit should be equal on both sides.
    i. The distance from the lateral border of the skull to the lateral margin of the foramen magnum should be equal on both sides.

35. Identify each lettered structure shown in Fig. 20-26.

A. _____

B. _____

C. _____

D. _____

E. _____

F. _____

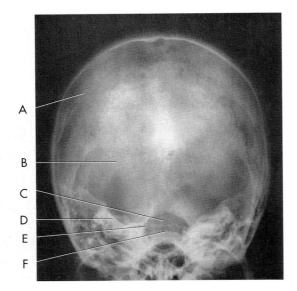

Fig. 20-26 AP axial skull (Towne method).

Items 36 through 43 pertain to the *PA axial projection (Haas method)*. Examine Fig. 20-27 as you answer the following items.

Fig. 20-27 PA axial skull (Haas method).

36. True or False. The PA axial projection (Haas method) demonstrates the occipital region of the cranium.

37. True or False. Hypersthenic patients should be positioned while recumbent in the supine position.

38. Which parts of the patient's head should be in contact with the table or vertical grid device?
    a. Chin and nose
    b. Chin and cheek
    c. Forehead and nose
    d. Forehead and cheek

39. In addition to the midsagittal plane, which positioning line of the skull should be perpendicular to the plane of the cassette?
    a. Orbitomeatal
    b. Glabellomeatal
    c. Acanthiomeatal
    d. Infraorbitomeatal

40. How many degrees and in which direction should the central ray be directed?

    a. 25 degrees caudad
    b. 25 degrees cephalad
    c. 30 degrees caudad
    d. 30 degrees cephalad

41. Where on the midsagittal plane of the patient's skull should the central ray enter?

    a. At the vertex of the skull
    b. At a point approximately $1\frac{1}{2}$ inches (4 cm) above the external occipital protuberance
    c. At a point approximately $1\frac{1}{2}$ inches (4 cm) below the external occipital protuberance
    d. At a point approximately 3 inches (7.5 cm) below the external occipital protuberance

42. From the list below, circle the four evaluation criteria that indicate the patient was properly positioned for the PA axial projection (Haas method).

    a. The entire cranium should be included.
    b. The orbital roofs should be superimposed.
    c. The petrous pyramids should be symmetric.
    d. The mandible should not overlap the cervical vertebrae
    e. The petrous pyramids should lie in the lower one third of the orbits.
    f. The mental protuberance should be superimposed over the anterior frontal bone.
    g. The dorsum sellae and posterior clinoid processes should be seen within the foramen magnum.
    h. The distance from the lateral border of the skull to the lateral border of the orbit should be equal on both sides.
    i. The distance from the lateral border of the skull to the lateral border of the foramen magnum should be equal on both sides.

43. Identify each lettered structure shown in Fig. 20-28.

    A. _____

    B. _____

    C. _____

    D. _____

    E. _____

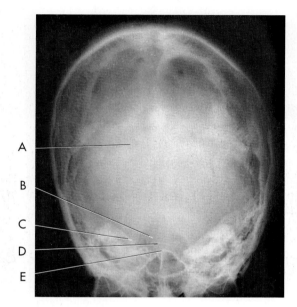

Fig. 20-28 PA axial skull (Haas method).

Items 44 through 50 pertain to the *submentovertical (SMV) projection*. Examine Fig. 20-29 as you answer the following items.

Fig. 20-29 Submentovertical cranial base.

44. Indicate how the midsagittal plane and the infraorbitomeatal line should be positioned—perpendicular or parallel—with reference to the plane of the cassette.

   a. Midsagittal plane: _____

   b. Infraorbitomeatal line: _____

45. To what positioning line of the skull should the perpendicular central ray be directed.

   _____

46. Describe where the central ray should enter the patient.

47. Through which cranial structure should the central ray pass?

   a. Sella turcica
   b. Ethmoidal air cells
   c. External acoustic meatus

48. From the list below, select the two positioning factors upon which the success of submentovertical projections most depend.

   a. Directing the central ray perpendicular to the OML
   b. Directing the central ray perpendicular to the IOML
   c. Directing the central ray perpendicular to the midsagittal plane
   d. Placing the OML as near as possible to parallel with the plane of the cassette
   e. Placing the IOML as near as possible to parallel with the plane of the cassette
   f. Placing the midsagittal plane as near as possible to parallel with the plane of the cassette

49. From the list below, circle the five evaluation criteria that indicate the patient was properly positioned for a submentovertical projection.

   a. The petrosae should be symmetric.
   b. The orbital roofs should be superimposed.
   c. The mandibular rami should be superimposed.
   d. The mental protuberance should superimpose the anterior frontal bone.
   e. The petrous pyramids should lie in the lower one third of the orbits.
   f. The mandibular condyles should be anterior to the petrous pyramids.
   g. The dorsum sellae should be seen and projected within the foramen magnum.
   h. The structures of the cranial base should be clearly visible as indicated by adequate penetration.
   i. The distance from the lateral border of the skull to the mandibular condyles should be equal on both sides.

50. Identify each lettered structure shown in Fig. 20-30.

A. _____

B. _____

C. _____

D. _____

E. _____

F. _____

G. _____

H. _____

I. _____

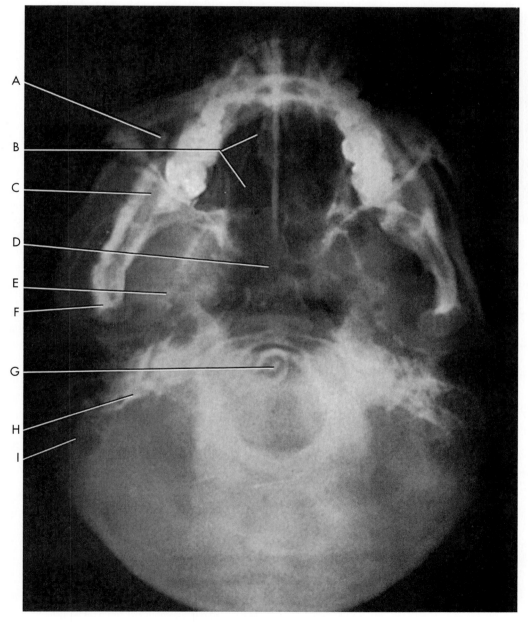

Fig. 20-30 Submentovertical cranial base.

Exercise 3: Positioning for the Sella Turcica

Instructions: To supplement computed tomography, a tightly collimated image of the sella turcica is often requested. This exercise pertains to the lateral projection of the sella turcica. Provide a short answer, select from a list, or identify structures for each item.

Examine Fig. 20-31 as you answer the following items about the *lateral projection for the sella turcica.*

Fig. 20-31 Lateral skull for the sella turcica.

1. Indicate how each of the following should be adjusted—perpendicular or parallel—to correctly position the patient for lateral projections of the sella turcica.

   a. Midsagittal plane: _____

   b. Interpupillary line: _____

   c. Infraorbitomeatal line: _____

2. Where exactly on the side of the head should the central ray enter?

3. What breathing instructions should be given to the patient?

4. From the list below, circle the four evaluation criteria that indicate the patient was properly positioned for a lateral projection of the sella turcica.

   a. The sella turcica should not be rotated or distorted.
   b. The anterior clinoid processes should be superimposed.
   c. The posterior clinoid processes should be superimposed.
   d. The sella turcica should be in the center of the radiograph.
   e. The petrous pyramids should lie in the lower one third of the orbits.
   f. The dorsum sellae should be seen and projected within the foramen magnum.
   g. The distance from the lateral border of the skull to the mandibular condyles should be equal on both sides.

5. Identify each lettered structure shown in Fig. 20-32.

A. _____

B. _____

C. _____

D. _____

E. _____

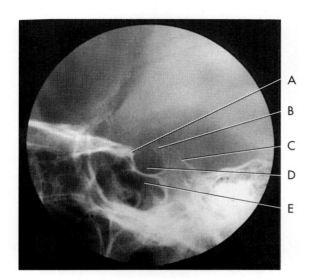

Fig. 20-32 Lateral sella turcica.

Exercise 4: Positioning for the Optic Canal and Foramen

Instructions: Parieto-orbital oblique projections and orbitoparietal oblique projections are two standard radiographic procedures used to demonstrate the orbital region, specifically the optic canal and foramen. This exercise pertains to those types of projections. Identify structures, select from a list, provide a short answer, or choose true or false (explaining any statement you believe to be false) for each item.

Items 1 through 10 pertain to the *parieto-orbital oblique projection (Rhese method)*. Examine Fig. 20-33 as you answer the following items.

Fig. 20-33 Parieto-orbital oblique projection (Rhese method).

1. In addition to the zygoma and nose, which other structure should be in contact with the x-ray table or vertical grid device?
   a. Ear
   b. Chin
   c. Forehead

2. Which positioning line of the head should be perpendicular to the plane of the cassette?
   a. Interpupillary
   b. Acanthiomeatal
   c. Infraorbitomeatal

3. Which body plane or positioning line should form an angle of 53 degrees with the plane of the cassette?
   a. Midsagittal plane
   b. Midcoronal plane
   c. Interpupillary line
   d. Acanthiomeatal line

4. True or False. Of the two orbits, the affected orbit should be placed closest to the cassette.

5. True or False. The patient should suspend respiration for the exposure.

6. True or False. The central ray should be directed caudally 15 degrees.

7. True or False. The parieto-orbital oblique projection demonstrates a cross-sectional view of the optic canal.

8. True or False. Incorrect angulation of the acanthiomeatal line will cause lateral deviation from the preferred location of the optic canal in the imaged orbit.

9. From the list below, circle the four evaluation criteria that indicates the patient was properly positioned for a parieto-orbital oblique projection.

a. The petrous ridges should be symmetric.
b. The entire orbital rim should be included.
c. The orbital roofs should be superimposed.
d. The dorsum sellae should be within the foramen magnum.
e. The supraorbital margins should lie in the same horizontal line.
f. The optic canal and foramen should be seen at the end of the sphenoid ridge.
g. The optic canal and foramen should lie in the inferior and lateral quadrant of the orbit.
h. The optic canal and foramen should lie in the superior and medial quadrant of the orbit.

10. Identify each lettered structure shown in Fig. 20-34.

A. _____

B. _____

C. _____

D. _____

E. _____

F. _____

G. _____

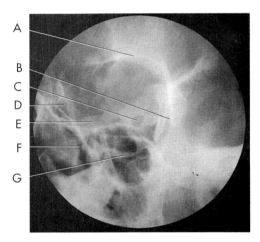

Fig. 20-34 Parieto-orbital oblique projection.

Items 11 through 20 pertain to the *orbitoparietal oblique projection (Rhese method).* Examine Fig. 20-35 as you answer the following items.

Fig. 20-35 Orbitoparietal oblique projection (Rhese method).

11. True or False. The patient should be positioned from either the seated (upright) position or the supine position.

12. True or False. Of the two orbits, the affected orbit should be placed farthest from the cassette.

13. True or False. The central ray should enter the affected orbit.

14. True or False. The orbitoparietal oblique projection causes less radiation exposure to the lens of the eye than the parieto-orbital oblique projection.

15. True or False. The orbitoparietal oblique projection results in more magnification of the orbit than the parieto-orbital oblique projection.

16. What positioning line of the head should be perpendicular to the cassette?

_____

17. What plane of the body should form an angle of 53 degrees with the cassette?

_____

18. How should the central ray be directed?
    a. Perpendicularly
    b. 53 degrees caudally
    c. 53 degrees cephalically

19. Which projection produces an image similar to that of the orbitoparietal oblique projection?
    a. Submentovertical projection
    b. Parieto-orbital oblique projection
    c. PA axial projection (Haas method)

20. From the list below, circle the four evaluation criteria that indicate the patient was properly positioned for an orbitoparietal oblique projection.
    a. The petrous ridges should be symmetric.
    b. The orbital roofs should be superimposed.
    c. The entire orbital rim should be included.
    d. The dorsum sellae should be within the foramen magnum.
    e. The supraorbital margins should lie in the same horizontal line.
    f. The optic canal and foramen should be seen at the end of the sphenoid ridge.
    g. The optic canal and foramen should lie in the inferior and lateral quadrant of the orbit.
    h. The optic canal and foramen should lie in the superior and medial quadrant of the orbit.

Exercise 5: Evaluating Radiographs of the Skull

Instructions: This exercise consists of radiographs of the skull, most of which show at least one positioning error, to give you some practice evaluating skull positioning. These images are not from *Merrill's Atlas of Radiographic Positions and Radiologic Procedures*. Examine each image and answer the questions that follow by providing a short answer.

1. Figs. 20-36 through 20-38 are lateral projection radiographs of a phantom skull. Only one image demonstrates acceptable positioning. Examine the images and answer the questions that follow. Refer to specific evaluation criteria for this projection when explaining your answers.

Fig. 20-36 Lateral skull.

Fig. 20-37 Lateral skull.

Fig. 20-38 Lateral skull.

a. Which image best demonstrates an optimally positioned skull? Explain.

b. Which image shows the skull incorrectly positioned because the vertex and midsagittal plane are tilted toward the plane of the cassette? Explain.

c. Which image shows the skull incorrectly positioned because the face and midsagittal plane are rotated toward the x-ray table and cassette? Explain.

d. Which image shows the skull positioned similarly to that seen in Fig. 20-17, Diagram *B*?

_____

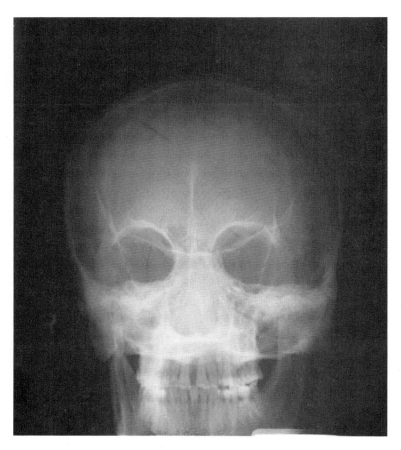

Fig. 20-39 PA skull showing incorrect positioning.

2. Fig. 20-39 shows a PA projection radiograph of a phantom skull with incorrect positioning. Examine the image and answer the questions that follow.

a. Assuming that the orbitomeatal line was perpendicular to the plane of the cassette, describe how the central ray most likely was directed.

c. What image characteristic most likely prevents this image from meeting all the evaluation criteria for this projection?

b. Describe where the petrous ridges should appear in the image when the central ray is directed caudally 15 degrees.

d. Describe the positioning error that most likely caused the image to appear as it does.

3. Fig. 20-40 shows a PA projection radiograph of a phantom skull with incorrect positioning. Examine the image and answer the questions that follow.

Fig. 20-40 PA skull showing incorrect positioning.

a. Assuming that the orbitomeatal line was perpendicular to the plane of the cassette, describe how the central ray most likely was directed.

b. Describe where the petrous ridges should appear in the image when the central ray is directed caudally 15 degrees.

c. Do the petrous ridges nearly fill the orbits?

_____

d. What image characteristic most likely prevents this image from meeting all evaluation criteria for this projection?

e. Describe the positioning error that most likely caused the image to appear as it does.

4. Figs. 20-41 and 20-42 show AP projection radiographs of a phantom skull. Only one image demonstrates acceptable positioning. Examine the images and answer the questions that follow.

Fig. 20-41 AP projection.

Fig. 20-42 AP projection.

a. Is the positioning quality for Fig. 20-41 acceptable or unacceptable?

_____

b. Is the positioning quality for Fig. 20-42 acceptable or unacceptable?

_____

c. Describe the positioning error that probably caused the unacceptable image.

d. Assuming that the orbitomeatal line was perpendicular for both images, in which way does the central ray appear to have been directed?

_____

5. Examine Fig. 20-43 and state why it does not meet the evaluation criteria for this type of projection.

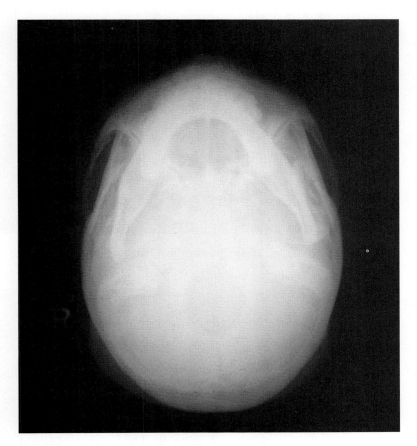

Fig. 20-43 Submentovertical projection showing incorrect positioning.

6. Figs. 20-44 through 20-46 are parieto-orbital oblique projection radiographs of a phantom skull. Only one image demonstrates the correct rotation of the head. Examine the images and answer the questions that follow. Refer to specific evaluation criteria for this projection when explaining your answers.

Fig. 20-44 Phantom skull orbit.

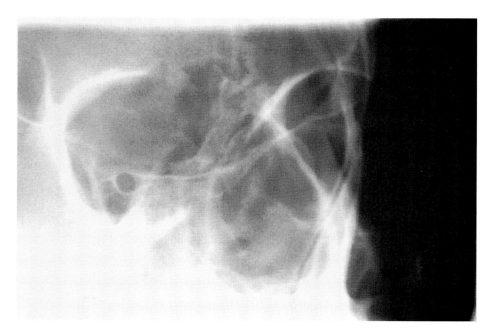

Fig. 20-45 Phantom skull orbit.

Fig. 20-46 Phantom skull orbit.

a. Which image best demonstrates ideal positioning of the phantom skull? Explain.

b. In which image does the midsagittal plane form an angle with the cassette that is considerably less than the required amount? Explain.

c. In which image does the midsagittal plane form an angle with the cassette that is somewhat greater than the required amount? Explain.

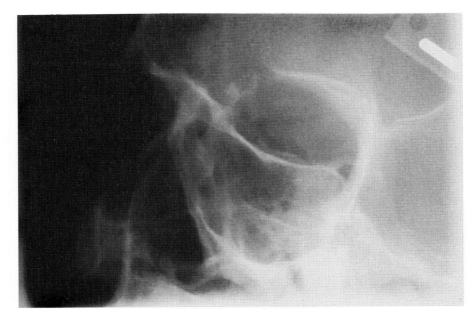

Fig. 20-47 Orbitoparietal oblique projection showing incorrect positioning of a phantom skull.

7. Fig. 20-47 is an orbitoparietal oblique projection radiograph of the left orbit of a phantom skull that is incorrectly aligned. Examine the image and answer the questions that follow.

a. What image characteristic indicates that the phantom skull was not correctly positioned?

b. What positioning error most likely produced this image?

c. How should the patient's position be adjusted to improve the demonstration of orbital structures with a subsequent radiograph?

Note to Students: Additional exercises referenced from Chapters 20 through 23 are found in the Appendix (Supplemental Exercises for Skull Positioning), which is located in this workbook. Students should complete the review exercises for those chapters before completing the appendix exercises.

Self-Test: Osteology and Radiography of the Skull

Instructions: Answer the following questions by selecting the best choice.

1. Which positioning line extends from the external acoustic meatus to the outer canthus?
   a. Orbitomeatal
   b. Glabellomeatal
   c. Acanthiomeatal
   d. Infraorbitomeatal

2. Which positioning landmark is located at the base of the nasal spine?
   a. Nasion
   b. Gonion
   c. Glabella
   d. Acanthion

3. Which positioning landmark is located at the most superior point of the nasal bones?
   a. Nasion
   b. Canthus
   c. Glabella
   d. Acanthion

4. Which positioning landmark is the smooth elevation that is located between the superciliary arches?
   a. Nasion
   b. Glabella
   c. Acanthion
   d. Mental point

5. Which positioning landmark is most superior?
   a. Nasion
   b. Gonion
   c. Glabella
   d. Acanthion

6. Where on the skull is the gonion located?
   a. Between the orbits
   b. On the anterior frontal bone
   c. On the posterior occipital bone
   d. On the lateroposterior part of the mandible

7. Where on the skull is the outer canthus located?
   a. Between the orbits
   b. At the mandibular angle
   c. Along each parietal eminence
   d. On the lateral border of each orbit

8. Which positioning landmark is located at the anterior portion of the mandible?
   a. Nasion
   b. Gonion
   c. Acanthion
   d. Mental point

9. Which suture articulates the frontal bone with both parietal bones?
   a. Sagittal
   b. Coronal
   c. Squamosal
   d. Lambdoidal

10. Which suture joins both parietal bones at the vertex of the skull?
    a. Sagittal
    b. Coronal
    c. Squamosal
    d. Lambdoidal

11. Which suture joins a parietal bone with both a sphenoid bone and a temporal bone?
    a. Sagittal
    b. Coronal
    c. Squamosal
    d. Lambdoidal

12. Which suture joins both parietal bones with the occipital bone?
    a. Sagittal
    b. Coronal
    c. Squamosal
    d. Lambdoidal

13. The bregma fontanel is located at the junction of which two sutures?
    a. Coronal and sagittal
    b. Coronal and squamosal
    c. Lambdoidal and sagittal
    d. Lambdoidal and squamosal

14. The lambda fontanel is located at the junction of which two sutures?
    a. Coronal and sagittal
    b. Coronal and squamosal
    c. Lambdoidal and sagittal
    d. Lambdoidal and squamosal

15. The bregma fontanel is located at the junction of which cranial bones?

    a. Frontal and both parietals
    b. Occipital and both parietals
    c. Frontal and sphenoid
    d. Occipital and sphenoid

16. The lambda fontanel is located at the junction of which cranial bones?

    a. Frontal and both parietals
    b. Occipital and both parietals
    c. Frontal and temporal
    d. Occipital and temporal

17. Which skull classification refers to a typical skull (in terms of width and length)?

    a. Mesocephalic
    b. Brachycephalic
    c. Dolichocephalic

18. Which skull classification refers to a long and narrow skull?

    a. Mesocephalic
    b. Brachycephalic
    c. Dolichocephalic

19. Which skull classification refers to a short and wide skull?

    a. Mesocephalic
    b. Brachycephalic
    c. Dolichocephalic

20. How many degrees is the angle formed between the midsagittal plane and the petrous pyramids in the mesocephalic skull?

    a. 36 degrees
    b. 40 degrees
    c. 47 degrees
    d. 54 degrees

21. How many degrees is the angle formed between the midsagittal plane and the petrous pyramids in the brachycephalic skull?

    a. 36 degrees
    b. 40 degrees
    c. 47 degrees
    d. 54 degrees

22. How many degrees is the angle formed between the midsagittal plane and the petrous pyramids in the dolichocephalic skull?

    a. 36 degrees
    b. 40 degrees
    c. 47 degrees
    d. 54 degrees

23. On which cranial bone are the superciliary arches located?

    a. Frontal
    b. Parietal
    c. Ethmoid
    d. Occipital

24. On which cranial bone is the cribriform plate located?

    a. Frontal
    b. Ethmoid
    c. Temporal
    d. Sphenoid

25. On which cranial bone is the crista galli located?

    a. Ethmoid
    b. Occipital
    c. Temporal
    d. Sphenoid

26. Which cranial bone has a petrous pyramid?

    a. Parietal
    b. Ethmoid
    c. Temporal
    d. Sphenoid

27. On which cranial bone is the sella turcica located?

    a. Frontal
    b. Ethmoid
    c. Temporal
    d. Sphenoid

28. Which cranial bone has the mastoid process?

    a. Parietal
    b. Ethmoid
    c. Temporal
    d. Sphenoid

29. On which cranial bone is the perpendicular plate located?

    a. Parietal
    b. Ethmoid
    c. Temporal
    d. Sphenoid

30. Which cranial bone has both greater and lesser wings?

    a. Ethmoid
    b. Occipital
    c. Temporal
    d. Sphenoid

31. With which cranial bone does the first cervical vertebra articulate?

    a. Ethmoid
    b. Occipital
    c. Temporal
    d. Sphenoid

32. The pterygoid processes project inferiorly from which cranial bone?

    a. Frontal
    b. Ethmoid
    c. Temporal
    d. Sphenoid

33. The foramen magnum is a part of which cranial bone?

    a. Frontal
    b. Occipital
    c. Temporal
    d. Sphenoid

34. From which cranial bone does the zygomatic process arise?

    a. Frontal
    b. Parietal
    c. Temporal
    d. Sphenoid

35. The external acoustic meatus is a part of which cranial bone?

    a. Frontal
    b. Parietal
    c. Temporal
    d. Sphenoid

36. The temporal process projects posteriorly from which facial bone?

    a. Vomer
    b. Maxilla
    c. Zygoma
    d. Temporal

37. Which bones comprise the bridge of the nose?

    a. Nasal
    b. Lacrimal
    c. Palatine
    d. Maxillae

38. With which bone does the mandible articulate?

    a. Hyoid
    b. Maxilla
    c. Zygoma
    d. Temporal

39. Where are the lacrimal bones located?

    a. Inside the nasal cavity
    b. On the lateral wall of each orbit
    c. On the medial wall of each orbit
    d. Inferior to the maxillary sinuses

40. Where is the vomer bone found?

    a. Posterior to the nasal bones
    b. On the floor of the nasal cavity
    c. On the lateral wall of the orbits
    d. In the posterior one fourth of the roof of the mouth

41. Which bone comprises most of the lateral wall of the orbital cavities?

    a. Maxilla
    b. Lacrimal
    c. Palatine
    d. Zygomatic

42. Which term refers to the anterior process of the mandibular ramus?

    a. Cornu
    b. Condyle
    c. Coracoid
    d. Coronoid

43. Which term refers to the posterior process of the mandibular ramus?

    a. Cornu
    b. Condyle
    c. Coracoid
    d. Coronoid

44. Which facial bones have alveolar processes?

    a. Vomer and mandible
    b. Vomer and zygomatic
    c. Maxillae and mandible
    d. Maxillae and zygomatic

45. Which bones form the posterior one fourth of the roof of the mouth?

    a. Maxillae
    b. Palatine
    c. Zygomatic
    d. Inferior nasal conchae

46. Which positioning landmark is located on the maxillae?

    a. Gonion
    b. Nasion
    c. Acanthion
    d. Mental point

47. Which two positioning lines or planes should be perpendicular to the cassette for the PA projection of the skull?

    a. Orbitomeatal line and midsagittal plane
    b. Orbitomeatal line and interpupillary line
    c. Infraorbitomeatal line and midsagittal plane
    d. Infraorbitomeatal line and interpupillary line

48. With reference to the patient, where should the cassette be centered for the PA projection of the skull?

    a. Nasion
    b. Glabella
    c. Acanthion
    d. Mental point

49. With reference to the patient, where should the cassette be centered for the lateral projection of the skull?

    a. Nasion
    b. External acoustic meatus
    c. 2 inches (5 cm) above the external acoustic meatus
    d. 2 inches (5 cm) below the external acoustic meatus

50. With reference to the cassette, how should the interpupillary line and the midsagittal plane be positioned for the lateral projection of the skull?

    a. Interpupillary line: parallel; midsagittal plane: parallel
    b. Interpupillary line: parallel; midsagittal plane: perpendicular
    c. Interpupillary line: perpendicular; midsagittal plane: parallel
    d. Interpupillary line: perpendicular; midsagittal plane: perpendicular

51. For the AP axial projection (Towne method) of the skull, how many degrees and in which direction should the central ray be directed when the orbitomeatal line is perpendicular to the cassette?

    a. 30 degrees caudad
    b. 30 degrees cephalad
    c. 37 degrees caudad
    d. 37 degrees cephalad

52. For the AP axial projection (Towne method) of the skull, how many degrees and in which direction should the central ray be directed when the infraorbitomeatal line is perpendicular to the cassette?

    a. 30 degrees caudad
    b. 30 degrees cephalad
    c. 37 degrees caudad
    d. 37 degrees cephalad

53. Which positioning line should be parallel with the cassette for the SMV projection of the skull?

    a. Orbitomeatal line
    b. Glabellomeatal line
    c. Acanthiomeatal line
    d. Infraorbitomeatal line

54. Which projection of the skull can be correctly performed with the central ray angled 37 degrees?

    a. AP axial (Towne method)
    b. PA axial (Haas method)
    c. PA axial (Caldwell method)
    d. Parieto-orbital oblique (Rhese method)

55. Which projection of the skull can be correctly performed with the central ray angled 15 degrees?

    a. Submentovertical
    b. AP axial (Towne method)
    c. PA axial (Haas method)
    d. PA axial (Caldwell method)

56. Which projection of the skull produces a full basal image of the cranium?

    a. Lateral
    b. AP axial (Towne method)
    c. PA with perpendicular central ray
    d. Submentovertical (Schüller method)

57. Which projection of the skull projects the petrous bones in the lower third of the orbits?

    a. PA axial (Haas method)
    b. AP axial (Towne method)
    c. PA axial (Caldwell method)
    d. PA with perpendicular central ray

58. Which projection of the skull should be obtained when the frontal bone is of primary interest?

    a. PA axial (Haas method)
    b. AP axial (Towne method)
    c. PA axial (Caldwell method)
    d. PA with perpendicular central ray

59. Which evaluation criterion pertains to the AP axial projection (Towne method) of the skull?

    a. The orbital roofs should be superimposed.
    b. The mental protuberance should superimpose the anterior frontal bone.
    c. Part of the sella turcica should be seen within the foramen magnum.
    d. The distance from the lateral border of the skull to the lateral border of the orbit should be the same on both sides.

60. Which evaluation criterion pertains to the PA projection of the skull?

    a. The orbital roofs should be superimposed.
    b. The mental protuberance should superimpose the anterior frontal bone.
    c. Part of the sella turcica should be seen within the foramen magnum.
    d. The distance from the lateral border of the skull to the lateral border of the orbit should be the same on both sides.

61. Which evaluation criterion pertains to the lateral projection of the skull?

    a. The orbital roofs should be superimposed.
    b. The mental protuberance should superimpose the anterior frontal bone.
    c. Part of the sella turcica should be seen within the foramen magnum.
    d. The distance from the lateral border of the skull to the lateral border of the orbit should be the same on both sides.

62. Which evaluation criterion pertains to the SMV projection of the skull?

    a. The orbital roofs should be superimposed.
    b. The mental protuberance should superimpose the anterior frontal bone.
    c. Part of the sella turcica should be seen within the foramen magnum.
    d. The distance from the lateral border of the skull to the lateral border of the orbit should be the same on both sides.

63. For the PA axial projection (Haas method) of the skull, where should the central ray enter the patient's head?

    a. Nasion
    b. Acanthion
    c. $1\frac{1}{2}$ inches (4 cm) above the external occipital protuberance
    d. $1\frac{1}{2}$ inches (4 cm) below the external occipital protuberance

64. How many degrees and in which direction should the central ray be directed for the PA axial projection (Haas method) of the skull?

    a. 15 degrees caudad
    b. 15 degrees cephalad
    c. 25 degrees caudad
    d. 25 degrees cephalad

65. For the parieto-orbital oblique projection (Rhese method) of the skull, which positioning line should be perpendicular to the cassette?

    a. Orbitomeatal
    b. Glabellomeatal
    c. Acanthiomeatal
    d. Infraorbitomeatal

66. For the orbitoparietal oblique projection (Rhese method) of the skull, which positioning line should be perpendicular to the cassette?

    a. Orbitomeatal
    b. Glabellomeatal
    c. Acanthiomeatal
    d. Infraorbitomeatal

67. With reference to the orbit, where should the optic foramen be imaged on the radiograph to indicate correct positioning of the patient for the parieto-orbital oblique projection (Rhese method) of the skull?

    a. Within the lower inner quadrant
    b. Within the lower outer quadrant
    c. Within the upper inner quadrant
    d. Within the upper outer quadrant

68. For the parieto-orbital oblique projection (Rhese method) of the skull, how many degrees should the angle be that is formed between the midsagittal plane and the cassette?

    a. 25 degrees
    b. 37 degrees
    c. 53 degrees
    d. 55 degrees

69. With reference to the cassette, how should the interpupillary line and the midsagittal plane be positioned for the lateral projection to demonstrate the sella turcica?

    a. Interpupillary line: parallel; midsagittal plane: parallel
    b. Interpupillary line: parallel; midsagittal plane: perpendicular
    c. Interpupillary line: perpendicular; midsagittal plane: parallel
    d. Interpupillary line: perpendicular; midsagittal plane: perpendicular

70. For the lateral projection to demonstrate the sella turcica, where should the central ray be directed?

    a. $\frac{3}{4}$ inch (2 cm) anterior and $\frac{3}{4}$ inch (2 cm) inferior to the external acoustic meatus
    b. $\frac{3}{4}$ inch (2 cm) anterior and $\frac{3}{4}$ inch (2 cm) superior to the external acoustic meatus
    c. $\frac{3}{4}$ inch (2 cm) posterior and $\frac{3}{4}$ inch (2 cm) inferior to the external acoustic meatus
    d. $\frac{3}{4}$ inch (2 cm) posterior and $\frac{3}{4}$ inch (2 cm) superior to the external acoustic meatus

If your school has access to Mosby's Radiographic Instructional Series on Anatomy, Positioning, and Procedures, review Unit 20 at this time. Your instructor may request that you respond to the series' exercises on paper. This unit covers the following essential projections:

Cranium
Lateral projections, right or left
Lateral (cross-table) projections, right or left
PA and PA axial projections, Caldwell method
AP and AP axial projections
AP axial projections, Towne method
PA axial projections, Haas method

Cranial base
Submentovertical projections, Schüller method

Sella turcica
Lateral projections, right or left

Optic canal: foramen
Parieto-orbital oblique projections, Rhese method
Orbitoparietal oblique projections, Rhese method

CHAPTER 21

Facial Bones

Radiography of the Facial Bones

Note to students: For a review of facial bone anatomy, see Chapter 20.

Exercise 1: Positioning for Facial Bones and Nasal Bones

Instructions: A standard radiographic series to demonstrate facial bones includes different projections that examine facial structures from different perspectives. Some projections commonly used are the lateral, the parietoacanthial (Waters method), and the acanthoparietal (reverse Waters method). Additionally, a lateral projection of the nasal bones is sometimes added to a facial bones series because nasal bones are sometimes affected when other facial bones are damaged by trauma. This exercise pertains to the projections of the facial bones and nasal bones. Identify structures, fill in missing words, select from a list, or provide a short answer for each item.

Items 1 through 9 pertain to *lateral projections of the facial bones*. Examine Fig. 21-1 as you answer the following items.

Fig. 21-1 Lateral facial bones.

1. The cassette should be placed in the cassette holder

   _____ (crosswise or lengthwise).

2. The plane of the head that should be parallel with the plane

   of the cassette is the _____ (midsagittal or midcoronal) plane.

3. Which positioning line of the head should be perpendicular to the cassette?
   a. Orbitomeatal
   b. Interpupillary
   c. Acanthiomeatal
   d. Infraorbitomeatal

4. Which positioning line of the head should be parallel with the transverse axis of the cassette?
   a. Orbitomeatal
   b. Interpupillary
   c. Acanthiomeatal
   d. Infraorbitomeatal

5. Which facial bone should be centered to the cassette?
   a. Nasal
   b. Maxilla
   c. Mandible
   d. Zygomatic

6. How should the central ray be directed to the patient—perpendicularly, angled cephalically, or angled caudally?

   _____

7. Where on the patient's face should the central ray be directed?

8. From the list below, circle the four evaluation criteria that indicate the patient was properly positioned for a lateral projection of the facial bones.

   a. The sella turcica should not be rotated.
   b. The orbital roofs should be superimposed.
   c. The sella turcica should be seen within the foramen magnum.
   d. The mandibular rami should be almost perfectly super-imposed.
   e. The petrous bones should lie in the lower one third of the orbit.
   f. The mental protuberance should be superimposed over anterior frontal bone
   g. All facial bones should be completely included with the zygomatic bone in the center.
   h. The distance from the lateral border of the skull to the lateral border of the orbit should be equal on both sides.

9. Identify each lettered structure shown in Fig. 21-2.

   A. _____

   B. _____

   C. _____

   D. _____

   E. _____

   F. _____

   G. _____

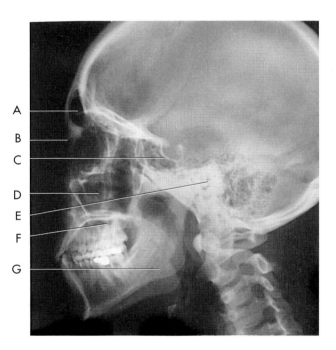

Fig. 21-2 Lateral facial bones.

Items 10 through 15 pertain to the *parietoacanthial projection (Waters method)*. Examine Fig. 21-3 as you answer the following items.

Fig. 21-3 Parietoacanthial facial bones (Waters method).

10. Indicate how the orbitomeatal line and the midsagittal plane should be positioned with reference to the cassette.

    a. Orbitomeatal line: _____

    b. Midsagittal plane: _____

11. To which landmark of the head should the cassette be centered?

    a. Nasion
    b. Acanthion
    c. Mental point
    d. Outer canthus

12. How should the central ray be directed relative to the cassette?

    a. Perpendicularly
    b. 37 degrees caudally
    c. 37 degrees cephalically

13. Describe where the petrous ridges most likely will appear in the image if the orbitomeatal line creates the following angles with the cassette:

    a. 25 degrees:

    _____

    _____

    b. 37 degrees:

    _____

    _____

    c. 55 degrees:

    _____

    _____

14. From the list below, circle the two evaluation criteria that indicate the patient was properly positioned for a parietoacanthial projection.

    a. The orbital roofs should be superimposed.
    b. The petrous ridges should nearly fill the orbits.
    c. The entire cranium should be demonstrated without rotation or tilt.
    d. The petrous ridges should be projected immediately below the maxillary sinuses.
    e. The distance between the lateral border of the skull and orbit should be equal on both sides.

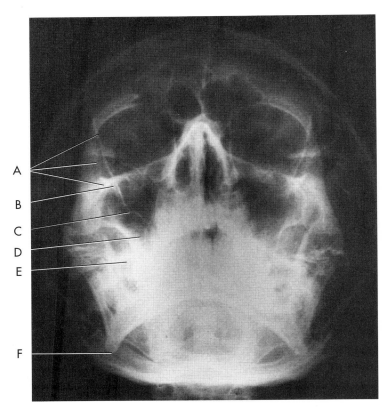

Fig. 21-4 Parietoacanthial facial bones (Waters method).

15. Identify each lettered structure shown in Fig. 21-4.

A. _____

B. _____

C. _____

D. _____

E. _____

F. _____

Items 16 through 24 pertain to the *acanthoparietal projection (reverse Waters method)*. Examine Fig. 21-5 as you answer the following items.

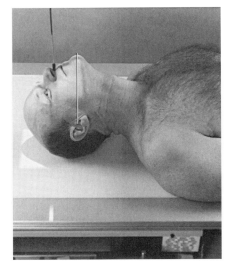

Fig. 21-5 Acanthoparietal facial bones (reverse Waters method).

16. The acanthoparietal projection can be used to demonstrate facial bones when the patient is lying in the

    _____ (prone or supine) position.

17. The image of the acanthoparietal projection is similar to

    the image of the _____ projection

    (_____ method).

18. Which plane and positioning line of the head should be perpendicular to the cassette?
    a. Midsagittal plane and orbitomeatal line
    b. Midsagittal plane and mentomeatal line
    c. Midcoronal plane and orbitomeatal line
    d. Midcoronal plane and mentomeatal line

19. Where should the midpoint of the cassette be centered to the patient?
    a. Nasion
    b. Glabella
    c. Acanthion
    d. 1 inch (2.5 cm) inferior to the acanthion

20. Which breathing instructions should be given to the patient?
    a. Stop breathing.
    b. Breathe slowly.
    c. Breathe rapidly.

21. How should the central ray be directed?
    a. Perpendicularly
    b. 15 degrees caudally
    c. 15 degrees cephalically
    d. 30 degrees cephalically

22. To which positioning landmark should the central ray be directed?
    a. Nasion
    b. Glabella
    c. Acanthion
    d. Mental point

23. From the list below, circle the two evaluation criteria that indicate the patient was properly positioned for an acanthoparietal projection (reverse Waters method).
    a. The orbital roofs should be superimposed.
    b. The petrous ridges should nearly fill the orbits.
    c. The petrous ridges should be projected in the maxillary sinuses.
    d. The petrous ridges should be projected immediately below the maxillary sinuses.
    e. The distance between the lateral border of the skull and orbit should be equal on both sides.

24. Identify each lettered structure shown in Fig. 21-6.

    A. _____

    B. _____

    C. _____

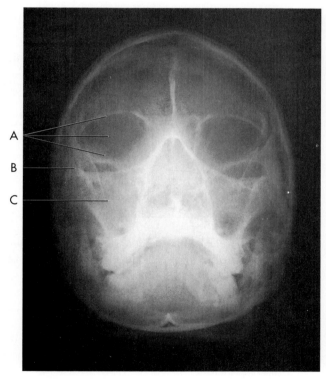

Fig. 21-6 Acanthoparietal facial bones (reverse Waters method).

Items 25 through 30 pertain to the *lateral projection of the nasal bones.* Examine Fig. 21-7 as you answer the following items.

Fig. 21-7 Lateral nasal bones.

25. Indicate how the interpupillary line and midsagittal plane should be positioned with reference to the cassette—perpendicular or parallel.

    a. Interpupillary line: _____

    b. Midsagittal plane: _____

26. How many exposures should be made on one cassette?

    _____

27. To which facial landmark—the nasion or acanthion—should the unmasked portion of the cassette should be centered?

    _____

28. Describe how and to where the central ray should be directed.

29. From the list below, circle the two evaluation criteria that indicate the patient was properly positioned for a lateral projection.

    a All facial bones should be demonstrated.
    b. The zygomatic processes should be seen superimposed.
    c. The anterior nasal spine and frontonasal suture should be visualized.
    d. The nasal bone and soft tissue should be demonstrated without rotation.

30. Identify each lettered structure shown in Fig. 21-8.

    A. _____ (suture)

    B. _____

    C. _____

Fig. 21-8 Lateral nasal bones.

Exercise 2: Positioning for Zygomatic Arches

Instructions: Zygomatic arches are commonly demonstrated with three projections: two slightly different tangential projections and an AP axial projection. This exercise pertains to those projections. Identify structures, fill in missing words, provide a short answer, select from a list, or choose true or false (explaining any statement you believe to be false) for each item.

Items 1 through 9 pertain to the *tangential projection for bilateral zygomatic arches*. Examine Fig. 21-9 as you answer the following items.

Fig. 21-9 Tangential zygomatic arches.

1. True or False. The tangential projection should demonstrate both zygomatic arches with one exposure.

2. True or False. Zygomatic arches should be demonstrated superimposed with the anterior frontal bone.

3. True or False. The entire cranial base should be demonstrated.

4. True or False. The midsagittal plane should be parallel with the cassette.

5. Which positioning line of the head should be parallel with the cassette?

   a. Orbitomeatal
   b. Acanthiomeatal
   c. Infraorbitomeatal

6. Which part of the patient should be in contact with the grid device?

   a. Forehead
   b. Mandible
   c. Vertex of the skull

7. Which statement best describes how the central ray should be directed?

   a. Angled cephalically and centered to the glabella
   b. Angled caudally and centered to the zygomatic arch of interest
   c. Perpendicular to the infraorbitomeatal line and centered on the midsagittal plane of the throat

8. For the tangential projection, what causes the zygomatic arches to be projected beyond the parietal eminences?

   a. The divergent x-ray beam
   b. The head tilted 15 degrees
   c. The head rotated 15 degrees

9. From the list below circle the three evaluation criteria that indicate the patient was properly positioned for the tangential projection.

   a. No rotation of the head should occur.
   b. The zygomatic arches should be free from overlying structures.
   c. The entire cranium should be demonstrated without rotation or tilt.
   d. The zygomatic arches should be symmetric and without foreshortening.
   e. The structures of the cranial base should be clearly visible as indicated by adequate penetration.
   f. The distance from the lateral border of the skull to the lateral border of the orbit should be equal on both sides.

Items 10 through 14 pertain to the *tangential projection*. Examine Fig. 21-10 as you answer the following items.

Fig. 21-10 Tangential zygomatic arch.

10. True or False. The patient should hyperextend his or her neck and rest his or her head on the vertex.

11. True or False. The midsagittal plane should be perpendicular to the cassette.

12. What positioning line of the head should be as parallel as possible with the cassette?

_____

13. Describe how the central ray should be directed.

14. From the list below, circle the evaluation criterion that indicates the patient was properly positioned for a tangential projection.
   a. No rotation of the head should occur.
   b. The zygomatic arch should be free from overlying structures.
   c. The entire cranium should be demonstrated without rotation or tilt.

Items 15 through 20 pertain to the *AP axial projection (modified Towne method)*. Examine Fig. 21-11 as you answer the following items.

Fig. 21-11 AP axial zygomatic arches (modified Towne method).

15. Indicate how the orbitomeatal line and midsagittal plane should be positioned with reference to the cassette—perpendicular or parallel.

   a. Orbitomeatal line: _____

   b. Midsagittal plane: _____

16. How many degrees and in which direction should the central ray be directed when each of the following positioning lines is placed perpendicular to the plane of the cassette?

   a. Orbitomeatal line: _____

   b. Infraorbitomeatal line: _____

17. The central ray should enter 1 inch (2.5 cm) above the

   landmark _____.

18. True or False. Both zygomatic arches should be demonstrated on the radiograph with a single exposure.

19. True or False. The entire vertex should be included on the radiograph.

20. Identify each lettered structure shown in Fig. 21-12.

A. _____

B. _____

C. _____

Fig. 21-12 AP axial zygomatic arches (modified Towne method).

Exercise 3: Positioning for the Mandible

Instructions: Usually three or four projections are needed to demonstrate the mandible. PA, PA axial, and axiolateral oblique projections are often included in the typical mandible examination. This exercise pertains to those projections. Identify structures, provide a short answer, select from a list, or choose true or false (explaining any statement you believe to be false) for each item.

Items 1 through 10 pertain to the *PA projection demonstrating the mandibular rami.* Examine Fig. 21-13 as you answer the following items.

Fig. 21-13 PA mandibular rami.

1. To demonstrate the mandibular rami with the PA projection, which two facial structures should be touching the vertical grid device?

   a. Nose and chin
   b. Forehead and nose
   c. Forehead and cheek

2. Which positioning line should be perpendicular to the plane of the cassette?

   a. Orbitomeatal
   b. Glabellomeatal
   c. Acanthiomeatal
   d. Infraorbitomeatal

3. How should the midsagittal plane be positioned with reference to the cassette—parallel or perpendicular?

4. What breathing instructions should be given to the patient?

5. Through which positioning landmark of the face should the central ray exit?

   a. Nasion
   b. Acanthion
   c. Mental point

6. How does the vertebral column affect the image?

   a. It superimposes mandibular rami.
   b. It superimposes the central part of the mandibular body.
   c. It increases the object-to-image receptor distance (OID) of the mandible.

7. True or False. The central ray should be directed perpendicularly to the midpoint of the cassette.

8. True or False. The PA projection demonstrates the mandibular body without bony superimpositioning.

9. From the list below, circle the two evaluation criteria that indicate the patient was properly positioned for the PA projection of the mandibular rami.

   a. The entire mandible should be included.
   b. The mandibular rami should be superimposed.
   c. The mandibular body and rami should be symmetric on both sides.
   d. The temporomandibular articulation should be seen lying anterior to the external acoustic meatus.

10. Identify each lettered structure and fracture shown in Fig. 21-14.

    A. _____

    B. _____

    C. _____

    D. _____

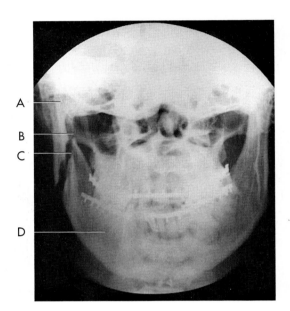

Fig. 21-14 PA mandibular rami.

Items 11 through 17 pertain to the *PA axial projection of the mandibular rami.* Examine Fig. 21-15 as you answer the following items.

Fig. 21-15 PA axial mandibular rami.

11. Which two facial structures should be touching the vertical grid device?

    a. Nose and chin
    b. Forehead and nose
    c. Forehead and cheek

12. Which body plane and positioning line should be perpendicular to the plane of the cassette?

    a. Midcoronal plane and orbitomeatal line
    b. Midcoronal plane and acanthiomeatal line
    c. Midsagittal plane and orbitomeatal line
    d. Midsagittal plane and acanthiomeatal line

13. Which breathing instructions should be given to the patient?

    a. Stop breathing.
    b. Breathe slowly.
    c. Breathe rapidly.

14. Which positioning landmark should be centered to the cassette?

    a. Nasion
    b. Glabella
    c. Acanthion
    d. Mental point

15. How many degrees and in which direction should the central ray be directed?

    a. 10 to 15 degrees caudad
    b. 10 to 15 degrees cephalad
    c. 20 to 25 degrees caudad
    d. 20 to 25 degrees cephalad

16. What prevents the central part of the mandibular body from being clearly demonstrated?

    a. Superimposition with the spine
    b. Caudal angulation of the central ray
    c. Increased object-to-image receptor distance

17. From the list below, circle the three evaluation criteria that indicate the patient was properly positioned for a PA axial projection.

    a. The entire mandible should be demonstrated.
    b. The mandibular rami should be superimposed.
    c. The condylar processes should be clearly demonstrated.
    d. The mandibular body and rami should be symmetric on both sides.
    e. The temporomandibular articulation should be seen lying anterior to the external acoustic meatus.

Items 18 through 31 pertain to axiolateral oblique projections of the mandible (with the patient either prone or upright). Figs. 21-16, 21-17, and 21-18 represent three upright axiolateral oblique projections that demonstrate parts of the mandible. Match each of the following positioning statements to one or more of these figures by writing the appropriate figure number in the space provided. Some statements may have more than one figure (projection) associated to them. Some statements do not relate to any of the three projections; answer "NA" for "not applicable" for these items.

Fig. 21-18 Upright axiolateral oblique projection.

Fig. 21-16 Upright axiolateral oblique projection.

Fig. 21-17 Upright axiolateral oblique projection.

_____ 18. Keep the head in a true lateral position.

_____ 19. Used for demonstrating the mandibular body.

_____ 20. Used for demonstrating the mandibular ramus.

_____ 21. Used for demonstrating the mental protuberance.

_____ 22. Rotate the head 30 degrees toward the cassette.

_____ 23. Rotate the head 45 degrees toward the cassette.

_____ 24. The central ray should exit the mental protuberance.

_____ 25. The central ray should be directed 15 degrees cephalad.

_____ 26. The central ray should be directed 25 degrees cephalad.

_____ 27. The central ray should be directed perpendicular to the cassette.

_____ 28. The orbitomeatal line should be perpendicular to the plane of the cassette.

_____ 29. The interpupillary line should be perpendicular to the plane of the cassette.

_____ 30. The broad surface of the ramus should be parallel with the plane of the cassette.

_____ 31. The broad surface of the mandibular body should be parallel with the plane of the cassette.

32. True or False. The mouth should be closed with the teeth held together.

33. True or False. The neck should be flexed to pull the chin downward.

34. True or False. The area of interest should be parallel with the cassette.

35. Identify each lettered structure shown in Fig. 21-19.

A. _____

B. _____

C. _____

D. _____

E. _____

F. _____

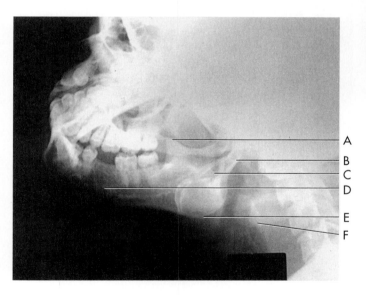

Fig. 21-19 Axiolateral oblique mandibular body.

Exercise 4: Positioning for the Temporomandibular Joints (TMJs)

Instructions: Two projections often performed to demonstrate temporomandibular joints are the AP axial projection and the axiolateral oblique projection. This exercise pertains to those projections. Identify structures, provide a short answer, select from a list, or choose true or false (explaining any statement you believe to be false) for each question.

Items 1 through 10 pertain to the *AP axial projection.* Examine Fig. 21-20 as you answer the following items.

Fig. 21-20 AP axial TMJs.

1. True or False. For the AP axial projection in the closed-mouth position, the upper posterior teeth should be in contact with the lower posterior teeth.

2. True or False. The long axis of the mandibular body should be parallel with the transverse axis of the cassette.

3. Why should the incisors *not* contact when the patient is positioned for the closed-mouth AP axial projection?

4. Identify a typical situation in which the patient should not be asked to open his or her mouth wide for an AP axial projection. Explain why.

5. Which plane and positioning line of the head should be perpendicular to the cassette?

   a. Midcoronal plane and orbitomeatal line
   b. Midcoronal plane and infraorbitomeatal line
   c. Midsagittal plane and orbitomeatal line
   d. Midsagittal plane and infraorbitomeatal line

6. How many degrees and in which direction should the central ray be directed?

   a. 25 degrees caudad
   b. 25 degrees cephalad
   c. 35 degrees caudad
   d. 35 degrees cephalad

7. Where should the central ray enter the patient?

   a. Glabella
   b. Acanthion
   c. 3 inches (7.5 cm) above the nasion
   d. 3 inches (7.5 cm) below the nasion

8. To which landmark should the cassette be centered?

   a. Nasion
   b. Glabella
   c. Central ray
   d. Mental protuberance

9. From the list below, circle the two evaluation criteria that indicate the patient was properly positioned for an AP axial projection with the mouth closed.

   a. The head should not be rotated.
   b. The condyle should be seen anterior to the external acoustic meatus.
   c. Only minimal superimposition by the petrosa on the condyle should be seen.
   d. The condyle and temporomandibular articulation should be seen below the pars petrosa.

10. From the list below, circle the two evaluation criteria that indicate the patient was properly positioned for an AP axial projection with the mouth open.

    a. The head should not be rotated.
    b. The condyle should be seen anterior to the external acoustic meatus.
    c. Only minimal superimposition by the petrosa on the condyle should be seen.
    d. The condyle and temporomandibular articulation should be demonstrated below the petrosa.

Items 11 through 20 pertain to *axiolateral oblique projections.* Examine Fig. 21-21 as you answer the following items.

Fig. 21-21 Axiolateral oblique TMJ.

11. Where on the patient should the cassette be centered?

    a. 2 inches (5 cm) inferior to the TMJs
    b. 2 inches (5 cm) superior to the TMJs
    c. ½ inch (1.2 cm) anterior to the external acoustic meatus
    d. ½ inch (1.2 cm) posterior to the external acoustic meatus

12. How should the midsagittal plane be positioned with reference to the cassette?

    a. Parallel
    b. Perpendicular
    c. Form an angle of 15 degrees
    d. form an angle of 37 degrees

13. Which positioning line of the head should be parallel with the transverse axis of the cassette?

    a. Orbitomeatal
    b. Interpupillary
    c. Acanthiomeatal
    d. Infraorbitomeatal

14. How many degrees and in what direction should the central ray be directed?

_____

15. Through what structure should the central ray exit the patient?

_____

16. In relation to surrounding structures, where in the image should the mandibular condyle be seen for axiolateral oblique projections with the patient holding the mouth closed?

_____

17. True or False. The central ray should enter the patient at the TMJ farther from the cassette.

18. True or False. Both open- and closed-mouth positions should be performed with the axiolateral oblique projection unless contraindicated.

19. True or False. The entire side of the mandible from the condyle to the symphysis should be demonstrated.

20. Identify each lettered structure shown in Fig. 21-22.

A. _____

B. _____

C. _____

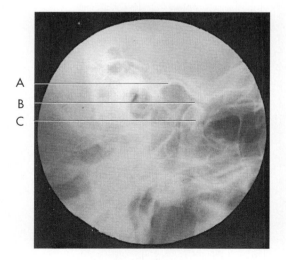

Fig. 21-22 Axiolateral oblique TMJ with the patient's mouth open.

Exercise 5: Evaluating Radiographs of Facial Bones

Instructions: This exercise consists of facial bone radiographs to give you some practice evaluating facial bone positioning. These images are not from _Merrill's Atlas of Radiographic Positions and Radiologic Procedures_. Most images show at least one positioning error. Examine each image and answer the questions that follow by providing a short answer.

1. Fig. 21-23 shows a lateral projection radiograph of the facial bones with incorrect positioning of a phantom skull. Examine the image and state why it does not meet the evaluation criteria for this type of projection.

Fig. 21-23 Lateral facial bones showing incorrect positioning of a phantom skull.

2. Figs. 21-24 through 21-26 show parietoacanthial projection radiographs of the facial bones of a phantom skull. Only one image demonstrates acceptable positioning. Examine the images and answer the questions that follow.

a. Which image demonstrates acceptable positioning?

_____

b. In which image does the phantom skull appear to be incorrectly positioned because the angle between the orbitomeatal line and the cassette is greater than the required amount? (This error results when the patient is unable to extend the neck far enough.)

_____

c. In which image does the phantom skull appear to be incorrectly positioned because the angle between the orbitomeatal line and the cassette is less than the required amount? (This error results when the patient extends the neck too much.)

_____

Fig. 21-25 Radiograph of a phantom skull positioned for the parietoacanthial projection.

Fig. 21-24 Radiograph of a phantom skull positioned for the parietoacanthial projection.

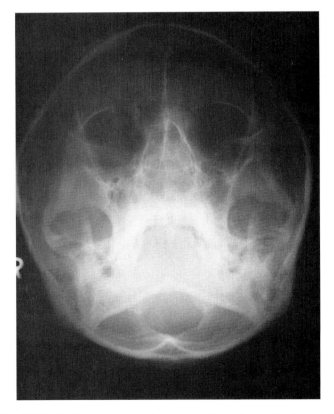

Fig. 21-26 Radiograph of a phantom skull positioned for the parietoacanthial projection.

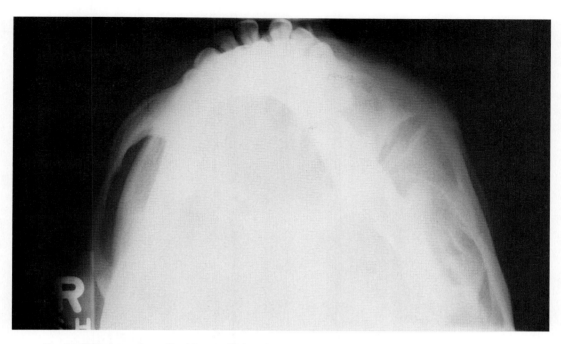

Fig. 21-27 Submentovertical-tangential projection of a phantom skull for zygomatic arches.

3. Fig. 21-27 shows a tangential projection radiograph of the zygomatic arches with incorrect positioning of a phantom skull. Examine the image and answer the questions that follow.

   a. What image characteristics prevent the image from meeting all evaluation criteria for this projection?

   b. What positioning error most likely resulted in this unacceptable image?

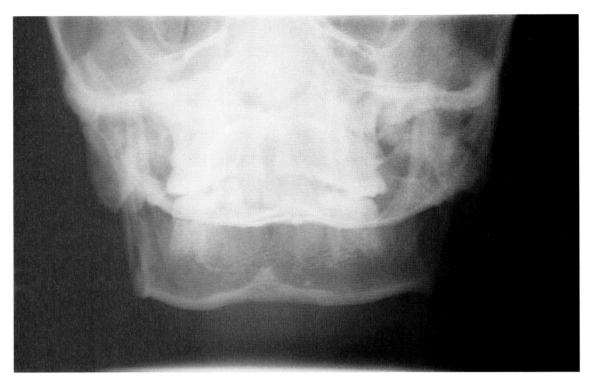

Fig. 21-28 PA mandibular rami showing incorrect positioning of a phantom skull.

4. Fig. 21-28 shows a PA projection radiograph demonstrating the mandibular rami with incorrect positioning of a phantom skull. Examine the image and answer the questions that follow.

   a. What image characteristic prevents this radiograph from being of acceptable quality?

   b. To comply with the evaluation criteria for this projection, how should the position of the phantom skull be adjusted for a subsequent radiograph?

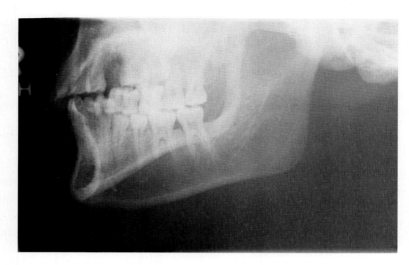

Fig. 21-29 Axiolateral oblique mandibular body showing incorrect positioning of a phantom skull.

5. Fig. 21-29 shows an axiolateral oblique projection radiograph of the mandibular body with incorrect positioning of a phantom skull. Examine the image and answer the questions that follow.

a. What image characteristic prevents the image from meeting all evaluation criteria for this type of projection?

b. How should the position of the phantom skull be adjusted for a subsequent radiograph?

Note to Students: Additional exercises referenced from Chapters 20 through 23 are found in the Appendix (Supplemental Exercises for Skull Positioning), which is located in this workbook. Students should complete the review exercises for those chapters before completing the appendix exercises.

Self-Test: Radiography of the Facial Bones

Instructions: Answer the following questions by selecting the best choice.

1. With reference to the patient, where should the central ray be directed for the lateral projection of the facial bones?

   a. Zygoma
   b. Nasal bones
   c. Outer canthus
   d. ¾ inch (2 cm) anterior and ¾ inch (2 cm) superior to the external acoustic meatus

2. With reference to the cassette, how should the central ray be directed for the parietoacanthial projection (Waters method)?

   a. Perpendicular
   b. 15 degrees caudad
   c. 23 degrees caudad
   d. 37 degrees caudad

3. Where should the petrous ridges be seen in the image of the parietoacanthial projection of the facial bones?

   a. Superior to the orbits
   b. Lower one third of the orbits
   c. Through the maxillary sinuses
   d. Below the maxillary sinuses

4. Which positioning line and angle indicate correct positioning of the head for the parietoacanthial projection (Waters method)?

   a. Orbitomeatal line; 37 degrees to the cassette
   b. Orbitomeatal line; perpendicular to the cassette
   c. Infraorbitomeatal line; 37 degrees to the cassette
   d. Infraorbitomeatal line; perpendicular to the cassette

5. Which evaluation criterion pertains to the parietoacanthial projection (Waters method)?

   a. The orbital roofs should be superimposed.
   b. The petrous ridges should be projected within the orbits.
   c. The zygomatic arches should be free from overlying structures.
   d. The petrous ridges should be projected immediately below the maxillary sinuses.

6. Which evaluation criterion pertains to the parietoacanthial projection (Waters method)?

   a. The orbital roofs should be superimposed.
   b. The zygomatic arches should be superimposed.
   c. The petrous pyramids should be projected within the orbits.
   d. The distance between the lateral border of the skull and orbit should be the same on both sides.

7. Which evaluation criterion pertains to the lateral projection of the facial bones?

   a. The orbital roofs should be superimposed.
   b. The petrous ridges should be projected within the orbits.
   c. The zygomatic arches should be free from overlying structures.
   d. The petrous ridges should be projected immediately below the maxillary sinuses.

8. Which evaluation criterion pertains to the tangential projection of the bilateral zygomatic arches?

   a. The orbital roofs should be superimposed.
   b. The zygomatic arches should be superimposed.
   c. The petrous ridges should be projected within the orbits.
   d. The zygomatic arches should be free from overlying structures.

9. An AP axial projection (modified Towne method) of the bilateral zygomatic arches produces an image similar to the AP axial projection (Towne method) of the skull. How many degrees and in what direction should the central ray be directed for this projection to demonstrate zygomatic arches when the OML is perpendicular to the cassette?

   a. 30 degrees caudad
   b. 37 degrees caudad
   c. 30 degrees cephalad
   d. 37 degrees cephalad

10. An AP axial projection (modified Towne method) of the bilateral zygomatic arches is performed similarly to the AP axial projection (Towne method) of the skull, except that the projection for the zygomatic arches requires that which of the following be done:

    a. The central ray should be directed cephalically.
    b. The central ray should be directed to the glabella.
    c. The orbitomeatal line forms an angle of 37 degrees with the cassette.
    d. The midsagittal plane forms an angle of 45 degrees with the cassette.

11. With reference to the cassette, how should the midsagittal plane be adjusted for the tangential projection demonstrating an individual zygomatic arch?

    a. Parallel with the cassette
    b. 15 degrees from perpendicular
    c. 37 degrees to the cassette
    d. 53 degrees to the cassette

12. To demonstrate the mandibular body with the axiolateral oblique projection, how should the patient's head be positioned?

    a. Keep the head in a true lateral position.
    b. From true lateral, rotate the head 15 degrees toward the cassette.
    c. From true lateral, rotate the head 30 degrees toward the cassette.
    d. From true lateral, rotate the head 45 degrees toward the cassette.

13. How many degrees and in which direction should the central ray be directed for the axiolateral oblique projection of the mandible?

    a. 15 degrees caudad
    b. 15 degrees cephalad
    c. 25 degrees caudad
    d. 25 degrees cephalad

14. Which projection is performed with the patient's head positioned true lateral and the central ray directed 25 degrees cephalad?

    a. Axiolateral oblique projections of the TMJs
    b. Axiolateral oblique projections of the mandible
    c. Parietoacanthial projections of the facial bones
    d. Tangential projections of the bilateral zygomatic arches

15. Which evaluation criterion pertains to the axiolateral oblique projection of the mandible?

    a. The mandibular rami should be superimposed.
    b. The opposite side of the mandible should not overlap the ramus.
    c. The mandibular condyles should be anterior to the petrous ridges.
    d. The mental protuberance should superimpose anterior frontal bone.

16. Which structure is of primary interest when the patient's head is rotated 15 degrees toward the cassette from a true lateral position and the central ray is directed 15 degrees caudad, entering about 1½ inches (4 cm) superior to the upside EAM?

    a. Orbit
    b. Mandible
    c. Zygomatic arch
    d. TMJ

17. Which of the following structures can be well demonstrated with an axiolateral oblique projection?

    a. Facial bones
    b. Zygomatic arches
    c. Maxillary sinuses
    d. TMJs

18. How many degrees and in which direction should the central ray be directed for the axiolateral oblique projection for TMJs?

    a. 15 degrees caudad
    b. 15 degrees cephalad
    c. 25 degrees caudad
    d. 25 degrees cephalad

19. For the AP axial projection of the TMJs, where should the central ray be directed?

    a. Nasion
    b. Glabella
    c. Acanthion
    d. 3 inches (7.5 cm) above the nasion

20. With reference to the patient, where should the cassette be centered for the axiolateral oblique projection of the TMJs?

    a. To the glabella
    b. ½ inch (1.2 cm) anterior to the external acoustic meatus
    c. 1 inch (2.5 cm) posterior to the external acoustic meatus
    d. 2 inches (5 cm) above the external acoustic meatus

If your school has access to Mosby's Radiographic Instructional Series on Anatomy, Positioning, and Procedures, review Unit 21 at this time. Your instructor may request that you respond to the series' exercises on paper. This unit covers the following essential projections:

Facial bones
   Lateral projections, right or left
   Parietoacanthial projections (Waters method)
   Acanthoparietal projections (reverse Waters method)
Nasal bones
   Lateral projections, right and left
Zygomatic arches
   Tangential projections
   Tangential projections (single arch)
   AP axial projections
Mandibular rami
   PA projections
   PA axial projections
Mandible
   Axiolateral oblique projections (prone)
   Axiolateral oblique projections (semisupine)
Temporomandibular articulations
   AP axial projections
   Axiolateral oblique projections, right and left

CHAPTER 22

Paranasal Sinuses

Review

Instructions: Usually three or four of the following projections comprise the typical paranasal sinus series: lateral, PA axial (Caldwell method), parietoacanthial (Waters method), submentovertical (SMV), and PA. This exercise pertains to the paranasal sinuses and the projections used to demonstrate them. Identify structures, provide a short answer, select from a list, or choose true or false (explaining any statement you believe to be false) for each item.

Items 1 through 10 pertain to the sinuses and radiographic procedures for the sinuses.

1. Name the four groups of sinuses.

2. Identify the sinus groups shown in Fig. 22-1.

   A. _____

   B. _____

   C. _____

   D. _____

Fig. 22-1 Two diagrams showing paranasal sinuses in relation to each other and surrounding structures: Diagram A shows the frontal view; Diagram B shows a lateral view.

3. Which paranasal sinus group is superior to the other sinus groups?

   a. Frontal
   b. Maxillary
   c. Ethmoidal
   d. Sphenoidal

4. Which paranasal sinuses are mostly located inferior to the orbits?

   a. Frontal
   b. Maxillary
   c. Ethmoidal
   d. Sphenoidal

5. Which paranasal sinuses are located directly below the sella turcica?

   a. Frontal
   b. Maxillary
   c. Ethmoidal
   d. Sphenoidal

6. Which paranasal sinus group is posterior to the ethmoidal sinuses?

   a. Frontal
   b. Maxillary
   c. Ethmoidal
   d. Sphenoidal

7. Which sinus group is subdivided into three main groups?

   a. Frontal
   b. Maxillary
   c. Ethmoidal
   d. Sphenoidal

8. In which body position should the patient be placed for radiographs of the paranasal sinuses?

   a. Prone
   b. Supine
   c. Upright

9. Give two reasons why the patient should be positioned as indicated in Question 8.

10. Why should the radiographer ensure that the exposure factors used do not cause the paranasal sinuses to appear underpenetrated?

Items 11 through 17 pertain to the *lateral projection.* Examine Fig. 22-2 as you answer the following items.

Fig. 22-2 Lateral sinuses.

11. State how the midsagittal plane and the interpupillary line should be placed with reference to the plane of the cassette—perpendicular or parallel.

    a. Midsagittal plane: _____

    b. Interpupillary line: _____

12. Where on the patient's head should the central ray be directed?
    a. 2 inches (5 cm) above the external acoustic meatus
    b. 2 inches (5 cm) below the external acoustic meatus
    c. ½ to 1 inch (1.2 to 2.5 cm) anterior to the outer canthus
    d. ½ to 1 inch (1.2 to 2.5 cm) posterior to the outer canthus

13. How should the central ray be directed relative to the patient's head?
    a. Perpendicular
    b. 15 degrees caudad
    c. 15 degrees cephalad

14. Which sinus group is of primary importance?
    a. Frontal
    b. Maxillary
    c. Ethmoidal
    d. Sphenoidal

15. How many sinus groups should be clearly demonstrated with lateral projection radiographs?
    a. One
    b. Two
    c. Three
    d. Four

16. From the list below, circle the six evaluation criteria that indicate the patient was properly positioned for a lateral projection.
    a. The sella turcica should not be rotated.
    b. The sinuses should be visualized clearly.
    c. The orbital roofs should be superimposed.
    d. All four sinus groups should be included.
    e. The mandibular rami should be superimposed.
    f. Close beam restriction of the sinus area is needed.
    g. The petrous ridges should be lying in the lower one third of the orbits.
    h. The anterior frontal bone should be superimposed by the mental protuberance.
    i. The petrous ridges should be lying just below the floor of the maxillary sinuses.
    j. The distance between the lateral border of the skull and the lateral border of the orbits should be equal.
    k. The distance from the lateral border of the skull to the mandibular condyles should be equal on both sides.

17. Identify each lettered structure shown in Fig. 22-3.

A. _____   D. _____

B. _____   E. _____

C. _____   F. _____

Fig. 22-3 Lateral sinuses.

Fig. 22-4 PA axial sinuses (Caldwell method). **A,** Cassette tilted 15 degrees. **B,** Same projection with a vertical cassette.

Items 18 through 25 pertain to the *PA axial projection (Caldwell method).* Examine Fig. 22-4 as you answer the following items.

18. What are the two ways for performing PA axial projections (Caldwell method)?
    a. Head tilt technique and head rotation technique
    b. Head tilt technique and vertical cassette technique
    c. Angled cassette technique and head rotation technique
    d. Angled cassette technique and vertical cassette technique

19. Regardless of which technique is used for performing the PA axial projection (Caldwell method), which of the following procedures is common for both techniques?
    a. Directing the central ray caudally
    b. Using a vertically placed cassette
    c. Centering the acanthion to the cassette
    d. Use of a horizontally directed central ray

20. How should the patient's head be positioned when the cassette is not vertical?
    a. With the orbitomeatal line parallel with the central ray
    b. With the infraorbitomeatal line parallel with the central ray
    c. With the orbitomeatal line perpendicular to the cassette
    d. With the infraorbitomeatal line perpendicular to the cassette

21. To which positioning landmark of the skull should the cassette be centered?
    a. Nasion
    b. Glabella
    c. Acanthion

22. Which sinus structures are primarily demonstrated?
    a. Frontal sinuses and anterior ethmoidal air cells
    b. Frontal sinuses and posterior ethmoidal air cells
    c. Maxillary sinuses and anterior ethmoidal air cells
    d. Maxillary sinuses and posterior ethmoidal air cells

23. Where should the petrous ridges be demonstrated in the image?
    a. Completely filling the orbits
    b. In the lower one third of the orbits
    c. Just below the floor of the maxillary sinuses

24. From the list below, circle the eight evaluation criteria that indicate the patient was properly positioned for a PA axial projection.
    a. The orbital roofs should be superimposed.
    b. The mandibular rami should be superimposed.
    c. The air-fluid levels, if present, are clearly visible.
    d. Close beam restriction of the sinus area is needed.
    e. The petrous ridges should be symmetric on both sides.
    f. All four sinus groups should be clearly demonstrated.
    g. The petrous ridges should lie in the lower one third of the orbits.
    h. The frontal and anterior ethmoidal sinuses should be visualized clearly.
    i. The anterior frontal bone should be superimposed by the mental protuberance.
    j. The petrous ridges should be lying just below the floor of the maxillary sinuses.
    k. The frontal sinuses should lie above the frontonasal suture and be clearly demonstrated.
    l. The anterior ethmoidal air cells above the petrous ridges should be clearly demonstrated.
    m. The distance between the lateral border of the skull and the lateral border of the orbits should be equal.

25. Identify each lettered structure shown in Fig. 22-5.

A. _____

B. _____

C. _____

D. _____

E. _____

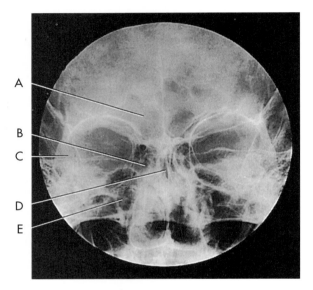

Fig. 22-5 PA axial sinuses.

Items 26 through 37 pertain to the *parietoacanthial projection (Waters method)*. Examine Fig. 22-6 as you answer the following items.

Fig. 22-6 Parietoacanthial sinuses, Waters method.

26. Which paranasal sinuses are best demonstrated with parietoacanthial projections (Waters method)?

_____

27. Where will the petrous ridges probably be demonstrated in the image if the patient does not sufficiently extend the neck?

28. How will the maxillary sinuses appear in the image—elongated or foreshortened—if the patient extends the neck too much?

_____

29. What positioning line of the head should form an angle of 37 degrees with the plane of the cassette?

_____

30. What positioning line of the head should be approximately perpendicular to the plane of the cassette?

_____

31. To what facial landmark should the cassette be centered?

_____

32. With reference to the surrounding structures, where should petrous ridges be demonstrated in the image?

33. Where on the image should the rotundum foramina be demonstrated?

34. True or False. The patient's nose and forehead should touch the vertical grid device.

35. True or False. The midsagittal plane should be perpendicular to the cassette.

36. From the list below, circle the five evaluation criteria that indicate the patient was properly positioned for a parietoacanthial projection (Waters method).

   a. The orbital roofs should be superimposed.
   b. The mandibular rami should be superimposed.
   c. The maxillary sinuses should be visualized clearly.
   d. The petrous ridges should completely fill the orbits.
   e. Close beam restriction of the sinus area is needed.
   f. The petrous ridges should be lying in the lower one third of the orbits.
   g. The orbits and maxillary sinuses should be symmetric on both sides.
   h. The sphenoidal sinuses should be seen projected through the open mouth.
   i. The anterior frontal bone should be superimposed by the mental protuberance.
   j. The petrous pyramids should lie immediately inferior to the floor of the maxillary sinuses.
   k. The distance from the lateral border of the skull to the lateral border of the orbit should be equal on both sides.

37. Identify each lettered structure shown in Fig. 22-7.

   A. _____

   B. _____

   C. _____

   D. _____

   E. _____

   F. _____

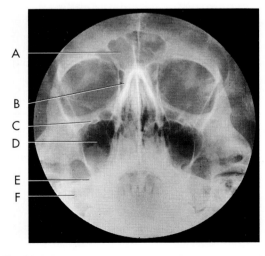

Fig. 22-7 Parietoacanthial sinuses (Waters method).

Items 38 through 42 pertain to the *parietoacanthial projection (open-mouth Waters method)*. Examine Fig. 22-8 as you answer the following items.

Fig. 22-8 Open-mouth parietoacanthial sinuses (Waters method).

38. To which landmark should the cassette be centered?

_____

39. What part of the patient's head should be resting on the vertical grid device?

_____

40. What positioning line of the skull should form an angle of 37 degrees with the plane of the cassette?

_____

41. Which of the sinuses should be demonstrated in the image through the patient's open mouth?

_____

42. From the list below, circle the six evaluation criteria that indicate the patient was properly positioned for a parieto-acanthial projection (open-mouth Waters method).

   a. The orbital roofs should be superimposed.
   b. The mandibular rami should be superimposed.
   c. The maxillary sinuses should be visualized clearly.
   d. The petrous ridges should completely fill the orbits.
   e. Close beam restriction of the sinus area is needed.
   f. The petrous ridges should be lying in the lower one third of the orbits.
   g. The orbits and maxillary sinuses should be symmetric on both sides.
   h. The sphenoidal sinuses should be seen projected through the open mouth.
   i. The anterior frontal bone should be superimposed by the mental protuberance.
   j. The petrous pyramids should lie immediately inferior to the floor of the maxillary sinuses.
   k. The distance from the lateral border of the skull to the lateral border of the orbit should be equal on both sides.

Items 43 through 55 pertain to the *submentovertical (SMV) projection*. Examine Fig. 22-9 as you answer the following items.

Fig. 22-9 Submentovertical sinuses.

43. True or False. The patient should rest his or her head with the chin contacting the vertical grid device.

44. True or False. The orbitomeatal line should be as close to parallel with the cassette as possible.

45. True or False. The midsagittal plane should be perpendicular to the cassette.

46. True or False. The central ray should be directed perpendicular to the IOML, entering the midline of the base of the skull so that it passes through the sella turcica.

47. True or False. The distance from the lateral border of the skull to the lateral border of the mandibular condyles should be the same on both sides.

48. True or False. The entire occipital bone should be included in the image of the SMV projection to demonstrate paranasal sinuses.

49. What two sinus groups should be well demonstrated with the SMV projection?

50. Where in the image should the mental protuberance appear in relation to the frontal bone?

51. Where in the image should the mandibular condyles appear in relation to the surrounding structures?

52. What positioning error most likely occurred if the mental protuberance is imaged posterior to, and separated from, the anterior frontal bone?

53. What positioning error most likely occurred if the mental protuberance is imaged superior to the anterior frontal bone?

54. From the list below, circle the three evaluation criteria that indicate the patient was properly positioned for an SMV projection.
    a. The orbital roofs should be superimposed.
    b. The mandibular rami should be superimposed.
    c. The maxillary sinuses should be visualized clearly.
    d. The mental protuberance should superimpose the anterior frontal bone.
    e. The mandibular condyles should be anterior to the petrous pyramids.
    f. The distance from the lateral border of the skull to the mandibular condyles should be equal on both sides.

55. Identify each lettered structure shown in Fig. 22-10.

A. _____

B. _____

C. _____

D. _____

E. _____

F. _____

G. _____

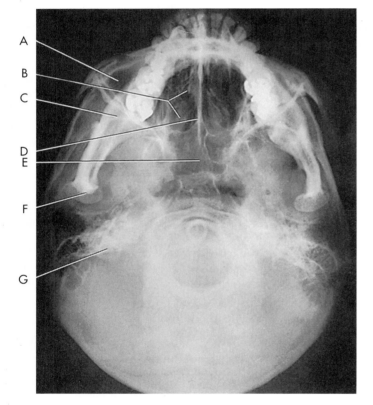

Fig. 22-10 Submentovertical sinuses.

Items 56 through 65 pertain to *PA projections.* Examine Fig. 22-11 as you answer the following items.

Fig. 22-11 PA posterior ethmoidal air cells.

56. True or False. The patient should be placed in the upright position.

57. True or False. The midsagittal plane should be perpendicular to the plane of the cassette.

58. True or False. The entire cranium should be included in the image for each PA projection of the sinuses.

59. True or False. The patient should be instructed to breathe slowly during the exposure to produce a suitable background density that will better demonstrate the maxillary sinuses.

60. Which positioning line of the head should be perpendicular to the plane of the cassette?
    a. Orbitomeatal
    b. Interpupillary
    c. Acanthiomeatal
    d. Infraorbitomeatal

61. Describe how and to where the central ray should be directed for PA projections demonstrating the following sinus groups.

   a. Posterior ethmoidal sinuses:

   _____

   _____

   b. Sphenoidal sinuses:

   _____

   _____

   c. Maxillary sinuses:

   _____

   _____

62. Where should the posterior ethmoidal sinuses be seen in the image of the PA projection of the posterior ethmoidal sinuses?
   a. Through the frontal bone
   b. Inferior to the base of the cranium
   c. Superior to the anterior ethmoidal air cells

63. Where should the sphenoidal sinuses be seen in the image of the PA projection of the sphenoidal sinuses?
   a. Through the frontal bone
   b. Inferior to the base of the cranium
   c. Superior to the anterior ethmoidal air cells

64. Where should the maxillary sinuses be seen in the image of the PA projection of the maxillary sinuses?
   a. Through the frontal bone
   b. Inferior to the base of the cranium
   c. Superior to the anterior ethmoidal air cells

65. From the list below, circle the three evaluation criteria that indicate the patient was properly positioned for all three PA projections of the sinuses.
   a. The orbital roofs should be superimposed.
   b. Close beam restriction of the sinus area is needed.
   c. The petrous pyramids should be symmetric on both sides.
   d. The mental protuberance should superimpose the anterior frontal bone.
   e. The mandibular condyles should be anterior to the petrous pyramids.
   f. The distance between the lateral border of the skull and the midsagittal plane should be equal on both sides.

Note to Students: Additional exercises referenced from Chapters 20 through 23 are found in the Appendix (Supplemental Exercises for Skull Positioning), which is located in this workbook. Students should complete the review exercises for those chapters before completing the appendix exercises.

Self-Test: Radiography of the Paranasal Sinuses

Instructions: Answer the following questions by selecting the best choice.

1. Which structures should always be radiographed with the patient in an upright position?

   a. Orbits
   b. Mastoids
   c. Zygomatic arches
   d. Paranasal sinuses

2. Which of the following is the only projection for paranasal sinuses that adequately demonstrates all four sinus groups?

   a. Lateral
   b. Submentovertical
   c. PA axial (Caldwell method)
   d. Parietoacanthial (Waters method)

3. With reference to the outer canthus, where should the central ray be directed for the lateral projections of the sinus?

   a. Inferior
   b. Superior
   c. Anterior
   d. Posterior

4. Which sinus group is of primary importance in the lateral projection of the sinuses?

   a. Frontal
   b. Maxillary
   c. Ethmoidal
   d. Sphenoidal

5. Which sinus groups are best demonstrated with the PA axial projection (Caldwell method)?

   a. Frontal and sphenoidal
   b. Frontal and anterior ethmoidal
   c. Maxillary and sphenoidal
   d. Maxillary and anterior ethmoidal

6. For the PA axial projection (Caldwell method) of the sinuses, which positioning line, in addition to the midsagittal plane, should be perpendicular to the cassette?

   a. Orbitomeatal
   b. Interpupillary
   c. Glabellomeatal
   d. Infraorbitomeatal

7. Where should petrous ridges be seen in the image of the PA axial projection (Caldwell method) of the sinuses?

   a. Superior to the orbits
   b. Lower one third of the orbits
   c. Through the maxillary sinuses
   d. Below the maxillary sinuses

8. Which positioning line should form an angle of 37 degrees with the cassette for the parietoacanthial projection (Waters method)?

   a. Orbitomeatal
   b. Glabellomeatal
   c. Acanthiomeatal
   d. Infraorbitomeatal

9. With reference to the cassette, how should the central ray be directed for the parietoacanthial projection (Waters method)?

   a. Perpendicular
   b. 15 degrees caudad
   c. 23 degrees caudad
   d. 37 degrees caudad

10. Which paranasal sinus group is best demonstrated with the parietoacanthial projection (Waters method)?

    a. Frontal
    b. Maxillary
    c. Ethmoidal
    d. Sphenoidal

11. Where should the petrous ridges be seen in the image of the parietoacanthial projection (Waters method) of the paranasal sinuses?

    a. Superior to the orbits
    b. Lower one third of the orbits
    c. Through the maxillary sinuses
    d. Below the maxillary sinuses

12. Where should the central ray exit the head for the parietoacanthial projection (Waters method)?

    a. Nasion
    b. Glabella
    c. Acanthion
    d. Mental point

13. Which sinus group is not well demonstrated in the image produced by the parietoacanthial projection (Waters method)?

    a. Frontal
    b. Maxillary
    c. Ethmoidal
    d. Sphenoidal

14. Which two paranasal sinus groups are better demonstrated with the SMV projection than are the other sinuses?

    a. Frontal and maxillary
    b. Frontal and sphenoidal
    c. Ethmoidal and maxillary
    d. Ethmoidal and sphenoidal

15. Which projection of the sinuses demonstrates a symmetric image of the anterior portion of the base of the skull?

    a. Lateral
    b. Submentovertical
    c. PA axial (Caldwell method)
    d. Parietoacanthial (Waters method)

16. In which projection of the sinuses is the cassette centered to the nasion?

    a. Lateral
    b. Submentovertical
    c. PA axial (Caldwell method)
    d. Parietoacanthial (Waters method)

17. In which projection of the sinuses is the mentomeatal line approximately perpendicular to the plane of the cassette?

    a. Lateral
    b. Submentovertical
    c. PA axial (Caldwell method)
    d. Parietoacanthial (Waters method)

18. In which projection of the sinuses must the OML form an angle of 15 degrees with the plane of the cassette?

    a. Lateral
    b. Submentovertical
    c. PA axial (Caldwell method)
    d. Parietoacanthial (Waters method)

19. Which evaluation criterion pertains to the lateral projection of the paranasal sinuses?

    a. All four sinus groups should be included.
    b. The petrous pyramids should lie in the lower one third of the orbits.
    c. The mental protuberance should superimpose the anterior frontal bone.
    d. The petrous pyramids should lie immediately below the floor of the maxillary sinuses.

20. Which evaluation criterion pertains to the lateral projection of the paranasal sinuses?

    a. The orbital roofs should be superimposed.
    b. The petrous ridges should lie in the lower one third of the orbits.
    c. The mandibular condyles should be anterior to the petrous ridges.
    d. The mental protuberance should superimpose the anterior frontal bone.

21. Which evaluation criterion pertains to the PA axial projection (Caldwell method) of the sinuses?

    a. All four sinus groups should be included.
    b. The frontal and ethmoidal sinuses should be seen.
    c. The mandibular condyles should be anterior to the petrous ridges.
    d. The petrous ridges should lie immediately below the floor of the maxillary sinuses.

22. Which evaluation criterion pertains to the PA axial projection (Caldwell method) for sinuses?

    a. Orbital roofs should be superimposed.
    b. Mandibular rami should be superimposed.
    c. Petrous ridges should lie in the lower one-third of the orbits.
    d. Petrous ridges should lie immediately below the floor of the maxillary sinuses.

23. Which evaluation criterion pertains to the parietoacanthial projection (Waters method) for paranasal sinuses?

    a. Mandibular rami should be superimposed.
    b. Petrous ridges should lie in the lower one-third of the orbits.
    c. Mental protuberance should superimpose anterior frontal bone.
    d. Petrous ridges should lie immediately below the floor of the maxillary sinuses.

24. Which evaluation criterion pertains to the submentovertical projection for paranasal sinuses?

    a. Mandibular rami should be superimposed.
    b. Frontal and ethmoidal sinuses should be clearly seen.
    c. Mental protuberance should superimpose anterior frontal bone.
    d. Petrous ridges should lie immediately below the floor of the maxillary sinuses.

25. Which evaluation criterion pertains to the submentovertical projection for sinuses?

    a. Petrous ridges should lie in the lower one-third of the orbits.
    b. Mandibular condyles should be anterior to the petrous ridges.
    c. Mandibular condyles should be posterior to the petrous ridges.
    d. Petrous ridges should lie immediately below the floor of the maxillary sinuses.

If your school has access to Mosby's Radiographic Instructional Series on Anatomy, Positioning, and Procedures, review Unit 22 at this time. Your instructor may request that you respond to the series' exercises on paper. This unit covers the following essential projections:

Paranasal sinuses
   Lateral projections, right or left
Frontal and anterior ethmoidal sinuses
   PA axial projections (Caldwell method)
Maxillary sinuses
   Parietoacanthial projections (Waters method with open-mouth modification)
Ethmoidal and sphenoidal sinuses
   SMV projections
Ethmoidal, sphenoidal, and maxillary sinuses
   PA projections

CHAPTER 23

Temporal Bone

Review

Note to students: For a review of the temporal bone anatomy, see Chapter 20.

Instructions: Although computed tomography (CT) is often used to image internal cranial structures, standard radiography is still employed in small medical facilities to demonstrate the mastoid processes and petrous portions. The axiolateral projections (modified Law method, single tube-angulation) can be used to image mastoid air cells, and both axiolateral oblique projections (Stenvers method, posterior profile, and Arcelin method, anterior profile) can be used to demonstrate petrous portions. This exercise pertains to those types of projections. Identify structures, provide a short answer, select from a list, or choose true or false (explaining any statement you believe to be false) for each item.

Items 1 through 11 pertain to the *axiolateral projection (modified Law method, single-tube angulation)*. Examine Fig. 23-1 as you answer the following items.

Fig. 23-1 Axiolateral petromastoid portion (modified Law method, single-tube angulation).

1. Describe how the patient's head should be positioned.

2. Which procedure should be performed to prevent soft-tissue structures from overlapping the mastoid process of interest?
   a. Tape the auricle of the ear forward.
   b. Angle the central ray 25 degrees caudad.
   c. Angle the central ray 25 degrees cephalad.
   d. Rotate the patient's head until the midsagittal plane forms an angle of 30 degrees with the plane of the cassette.

3. If the patient is rotated 15 degrees from the right lateral position, which mastoid—right or left—is of interest? Is it the side closer to or farther from the cassette?
   a. Left side; closer to
   b. Left side; farther from
   c. Right side; closer to
   d. Right side; farther from

4. Where should the cassette be centered to the patient?
   a. 2 inches (5 cm) above the external acoustic meatus
   b. 2 inches (5 cm) below the external acoustic meatus
   c. 1 inch (2.5 cm) anterior to the external acoustic meatus of the side adjacent to the cassette
   d. 1 inch (2.5 cm) posterior to the external acoustic meatus of the side adjacent to the cassette

5. How many degrees and in what direction should the central ray be directed?

6. Where should the central ray enter the patient?

7. True or False. The patient's head should be placed and kept in the true lateral position.

8. True or False. The patient's head should be rotated from the true AP position until the midsagittal plane forms an angle of 15 degrees from vertical.

9. True or False. The interpupillary line should remain perpendicular to the cassette throughout the positioning procedure.

10. From the list below, circle the six evaluation criteria that indicate the patient was properly positioned for an axiolateral projection (modified Law method, single tube-angulation).

   a. Close beam restriction of the mastoid region is needed.
   b. The auricle of the ear should not superimpose the mastoid.
   c. The entire side of the cranium should be clearly demonstrated.
   d. The petrous ridges should superimpose the mastoid of interest.
   e. The mastoid process should be in profile below the margin of the cranium.
   f. The internal and external acoustic meatuses should be superimposed.
   g. The temporomandibular joint should be visualized anterior to the mastoid.
   h. The temporomandibular joint should be visualized posterior to the mastoid.
   i. The opposite mastoid should not superimpose but should lie inferior and slightly anterior to the mastoid of interest.
   j. The mastoid closer to the cassette should be included, and the air cells should be demonstrated and centered to the cassette.

11. Identify each lettered structure shown in Fig. 23-2.

A. _____   C. _____

B. _____   D. _____

Fig. 23-2 Axiolateral petromastoid portion (modified Law method).

Items 12 through 18 pertain to the *axiolateral oblique projection (Stenvers method, posterior profile)*. Examine Fig. 23-3 as you answer the following items.

Fig. 23-3 Axiolateral oblique petromastoid portion (Stenvers method), posterior profile.

12. What three points of the face should be in contact with the x-ray table or vertical grid device?

13. How many degrees and in what direction should the central ray be directed?

14. Where on the head should the central ray enter the patient?
    a. 2 inches (5 cm) above the external acoustic meatus
    b. 2 inches (5 cm) below the external acoustic meatus
    c. 3 to 4 inches (7 to 10 cm) anterior, and ½ inch (1.2 cm) superior to the upside EAM
    d. 3 to 4 inches (7 to 10 cm) posterior, and ½ inch (1.2 cm) inferior to the upside EAM

15. An angle of how many degrees should be formed by the midsagittal plane with the plane of the cassette?
    a. 15 degrees
    b. 37 degrees
    c. 45 degrees
    d. 53 degrees

16. Which positioning line of the head should be parallel with the transverse axis of the cassette?
    a. Orbitomeatal
    b. Interpupillary
    c. Acanthiomeatal
    d. Infraorbitomeatal

17. Which petrous pyramid is demonstrated in profile when the patient is facing toward the left shoulder? Is it the petrous pyramid closer to or farther from the cassette?
    a. Left side; closer to
    b. Left side; farther from
    c. Right side; closer to
    d. Right side; farther from

18. Identify each lettered structure shown in Fig. 23-4.

A. _____   D. _____

B. _____   E. _____

C. _____   F. _____

Fig. 23-4 Axiolateral oblique petromastoid portion (Stenvers method), posterior profile.

Items 19 through 25 pertain to the *axiolateral oblique projection (Arcelin method, anterior profile)*. Examine Fig. 23-5 as you answer the following items.

Fig. 23-5 Axiolateral oblique petromastoid portion (Arcelin method), anterior profile.

19. True or False. The patient should be placed in the supine position.

20. True or False. The midsagittal plane should be perpendicular to the cassette.

21. True or False. The infraorbitomeatal line should be perpendicular to the cassette.

22. How many degrees and in what direction should the central ray be directed?

23. Where should the central ray enter the patient?

24. Which petrous pyramid—right or left—is demonstrated in profile when the patient is facing toward the left shoulder? Is it the petrous pyramid closer to or farther from the cassette?

   a. Left side; closer to
   b. Left side; farther from
   c. Right side; closer to
   d. Right side; farther from

25. From the list below, circle the six evaluation criteria that indicate the patient was properly positioned for either a posterior profile projection (Stenvers method) or an anterior profile projection (Arcelin method).

   a. The petrous ridges should completely fill the orbits.
   b. The petromastoid portion should be demonstrated in profile.
   c. The entire side of the cranium should be clearly demonstrated.
   d. The internal and external acoustic meatuses should be superimposed.
   e. The lateral border of the skull to the lateral border of the orbit should be included.
   f. The mastoid should be demonstrated in profile below the margin of the cranium.
   g. The mandibular condyle should be projected over the first cervical vertebra near the petrosa.
   h. The posterior surface of the ramus should parallel or superimpose the lateral surface of the cervical vertebrae.
   i. The opposite mastoid should not superimpose, but should lie inferior and slightly anterior to, the mastoid of interest.
   j. The petrous ridge should lie horizontally and at a point approximately two thirds of the way up the lateral border of the orbit.
   k. The mastoid closer to the cassette should be included, with the air cells demonstrated and centered to the cassette.

   Note to Students: Additional exercises referenced from Chapters 20 through 23 are found in the Appendix (Supplemental Exercises for Skull Positioning), which is located in this workbook. Students should complete the review exercises for those chapters before completing the appendix exercises.

Self-Test: Radiography of the Temporal Bone

Instructions: Answer the following questions by selecting the best choice.

1. Which projection method produces an axiolateral view of a mastoid?
   a. Waters method
   b. Arcelin method
   c. Stenvers method
   d. Modified Law method

2. Which projection requires that the central ray be directed 15 degrees caudad?
   a. Parietoacanthial (Waters method)
   b. Axiolateral oblique (Arcelin method, anterior profile)
   c. Axiolateral oblique (Stenvers method, posterior profile)
   d. Axiolateral (modified Law method, single-tube angulation)

3. Which projection requires that the patient's head be rotated from true lateral, moving the face closer to the cassette, until the midsagittal plane forms an angle of 15 degrees with the cassette?
   a. Parietoacanthial (Waters method)
   b. Axiolateral oblique (Arcelin method, anterior profile)
   c. Axiolateral oblique (Stenvers method, posterior profile)
   d. Axiolateral (modified Law method, single-tube angulation)

4. Which projection requires that the central ray enter at a point 2 inches (5 cm) posterior to, and 2 inches (5 cm) superior to, the uppermost external acoustic meatus?
   a. Parietoacanthial (Waters method)
   b. Axiolateral oblique (Arcelin method, anterior profile)
   c. Axiolateral oblique (Stenvers method, posterior profile)
   d. Axiolateral (modified Law method, single-tube angulation)

5. For axiolateral projections (modified Law method, single-tube angulation), how many degrees and in which direction should the central ray be directed?
   a. 10 degrees caudad
   b. 10 degrees cephalad
   c. 15 degrees caudad
   d. 15 degrees cephalad

6. Which structure is best demonstrated when the patient's head is rotated from true left lateral, moving the face closer to the cassette until the midsagittal plane forms an angle of 15 degrees with the plane of the cassette, and the central ray is directed caudally to exit the skull 1 inch (2.5 cm) posterior to the external acoustic meatus?
   a. Left petrous portion
   b. Right petrous portion
   c. Left mastoid air cells
   d. Right mastoid air cells

7. If the patient is rotated 15 degrees from the left lateral position when performing the axiolateral projection (modified Law method, single-tube angulation), which mastoid is of interest? Is it the side closer to or farther from the cassette?
   a. Left side; closer to
   b. Left side; farther from
   c. Right side; closer to
   d. Right side; farther from

8. Which evaluation criterion pertains to the axiolateral projection (modified Law method, single tube-angulation)?
   a. The petrous ridges should lie in the lower one third of both orbits.
   b. The petrous ridges should be demonstrated in profile without distortion.
   c. The mastoid process should be projected below the shadow of the occipital bone.
   d. The mastoid closer to the cassette should be included, with the air cells demonstrated and centered to the cassette.

9. How many degrees and in which direction should the central ray be directed for axiolateral oblique projections (Stenvers method, posterior profile)?
   a. 10 degrees caudad
   b. 10 degrees cephalad
   c. 12 degrees caudad
   d. 12 degrees cephalad

10. How many degrees and in which direction should the central ray be directed for axiolateral oblique projections (Arcelin method, anterior profile)?
   a. 10 degrees caudad
   b. 10 degrees cephalad
   c. 12 degrees caudad
   d. 12 degrees cephalad

11. Which evaluation criterion pertains to the axiolateral oblique projection (Stenvers method, posterior profile)?

    a. The petrous ridge should lie in the lower one third of the orbit.

    b. The petromastoid portion should be demonstrated in profile without distortion.

    c. The mastoid process should be projected below the shadow of the occipital bone.

    d. The mastoid closer to the cassette should be included, with the air cells demonstrated and centered to the cassette.

12. Which projection requires that the patient's head be rotated from the PA position until the midsagittal plane forms an angle of 45 degrees with the cassette, and that the central ray be directed to exit the skull 1 inch (2.5 cm) anterior to the external acoustic meatus?

    a. Tangential for individual zygomatic arches

    b. Axiolateral oblique (Arcelin method, anterior profile)

    c. Axiolateral oblique (Stenvers method, posterior profile)

    d. Axiolateral (modified Law method, single-tube angulation)

13. Which projection requires that the patient's head be rotated from the AP position until the midsagittal plane forms an angle of 45 degrees with the plane of the cassette and that the central ray be directed to enter the side of the face at a point about 1 inch (2.5 cm) anterior and ¾ inch (2 cm) superior to the external acoustic meatus?

    a. SMV (Schüller method)

    b. Axiolateral oblique (Arcelin method, anterior profile)

    c. Axiolateral oblique (Stenvers method, posterior profile)

    d. Axiolateral (modified Law method, single-tube angulation)

14. Which structure is best demonstrated when the patient's head is rotated from the PA position, moving the occipital bone closer to the right shoulder, until the midsagittal plane forms an angle of 45 degrees with the plane of the cassette, and the central ray is directed to exit the skull 1 inch (2.5 cm) anterior to the external acoustic meatus?

    a. Left petrous portion

    b. Right petrous portion

    c. Left mastoid air cells

    d. Right mastoid air cells

15. Which structure is best demonstrated when the patient's head is rotated from the AP position, moving the face toward the right shoulder, until the midsagittal plane forms an angle of 45 degrees with the plane of the cassette, and the central ray is directed to enter the side of the face about 1 inch (2.5 cm) anterior and ¾ inch (2 cm) superior to the external acoustic meatus?

    a. Left petrous portion

    b. Right petrous portion

    c. Left mastoid air cells

    d. Right mastoid air cells

 If your school has access to Mosby's Radiographic Instructional Series on Anatomy, Positioning, and Procedures, review Unit 23 at this time. Your instructor may request that you respond to the series' exercises on paper. This unit covers the following essential projections:

Petromastoid portion
   Axiolateral projections (modified Law method, single-tube angulation)
   Axiolateral oblique projections (Stenvers method, posterior profile)
   Axiolateral oblique projections (Arcelin method, anterior profile)

CHAPTER 24

Mammography

SECTION 1

Anatomy and Physiology of the Breast

Instructions: Radiographers who perform mammography need to know the anatomy of the breast. This exercise pertains to the breast. Identify structures or fill in missing words for each item.

1. Identify each lettered structure shown in Fig. 24-1.

   A. _____

   B. _____

   C. _____

   D. _____

2. Identify each lettered structure shown in Fig. 24-2.

   A. _____

   B. _____

   C. _____

   D. _____

   E. _____

   F. _____

   G. _____

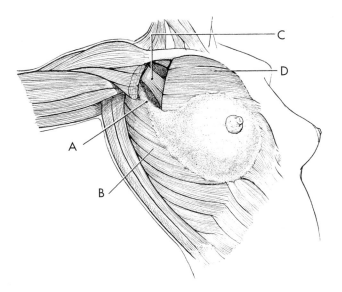

Fig. 24-1 Relationship of the breast to the chest wall.

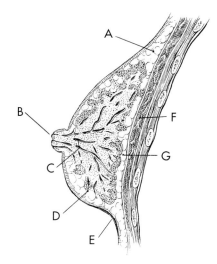

Fig. 24-2 Sagittal section through the breast illustrating structural anatomy.

3. The female breast functions as an accessory gland to the reproductive system by producing and secreting

   _____.

4. Another term for the female breast is the

   _____ gland.

5. The circular area of pigmented skin that surrounds the

   nipple is the _____.

6. The adult female breast contains _____ to _____ lobes.

7. The glandular elements found in the lobules of the female

   breast are the _____.

8. As a female gets older, the size of her breast lobules be-

   comes _____.

9. The normal process of change in breast tissues that occurs

   as the patient ages is termed _____.

10. Normal involution replaces glandular and parenchymal tissues with increased amounts of

    _____.

11. The ducts that drain milk from the lobes are the

    _____ ducts.

12. The axillary prolongation of the breast is also called the

    _____ of the breast.

13. Another term for the suspensory ligaments of the breast is

    _____ ligaments.

14. Approximately 75% of the lymph drainage is toward the

    _____.

15. The internal mammary lymph nodes are situated behind

    the _____.

SECTION 2

Radiography of the Breast

Exercise 1

Instructions: Breast radiography, or mammography, is employed to demonstrate diseases of the breast. This exercise pertains to mammographic procedures. Provide a short answer or select from a list for each question.

1. Why should the breast be bared for the examination?

2. Why should the patient remove deodorant and powder from the axilla?

3. Name the two standard projections routinely performed to demonstrate the breast.

4. What condition requires that a nipple marker be placed on the patient?

5. What procedure should a radiographer perform to help produce uniform breast thickness?

6. What procedure should a radiographer perform to identify the location of a palpable mass?

7. Why should the posterior nipple line be measured and compared between two projections?

8. Between what two structures should the posterior nipple line be measured in craniocaudal projections?

9. What is the maximum difference for the length of the posterior nipple line when comparing images of craniocaudal and mediolateral oblique projections?

10. Between examinations, what should a radiographer do to the image receptor surface and face guard?

Exercise 2

Items 1 through 10 are statements that refer to mammography positioning procedures. Examine each statement in Column A and identify the mammographic projection from Column B that most closely relates to the statement. Some statements pertain to more than one projection.

Column A

_____ 1. The breast should be perpendicular to the chest wall.

_____ 2. Slowly apply compression until the breast feels taut.

_____ 3. Elevate the inframammary fold to its maximum height.

_____ 4. Direct the central ray perpendicular to the base of the breast.

_____ 5. Direct the central ray 5 degrees mediolaterally to the base of the breast.

_____ 6. Instruct the patient to stand or be seated facing the image receptor holder.

_____ 7. Rotate the C-arm to direct the central ray to the medial side of the breast.

_____ 8. Adjust the height of the image receptor to the level of the inferior surface of the breast.

_____ 9. Adjust the height of the image receptor so that the superior border is level with the axilla.

_____ 10. Pull the breast tissue superiorly and anteriorly, ensuring that the lateral rib margin is firmly pressed against the image receptor.

Column B

a. Mediolateral

b. Craniocaudal

c. Mediolateral oblique

d. Exaggerated craniocaudal

Self-Test: Mammography

Instructions: Answer the following questions by selecting the best choice.

1. The lymphatic vessels of the breast drain laterally into which of the following lymph nodes?

    a. Axillary
    b. Thoracic
    c. Abdominal
    d. Internal mammary chain

2. Where is the tail of the breast located?

    a. Adjacent to the nipple
    b. Along the lateral side to the axilla
    c. Along the medial aspect of the breast
    d. In the glandular tissue against the chest wall

3. Which ducts drain milk from the lobes of the breast?

    a. Axillary
    b. Thoracic
    c. Lymphatic
    d. Lactiferous

4. How do breast tissues change after involution?

    a. Glandular tissues become dense and opaque.
    b. Fatty tissues are replaced with glandular tissues.
    c. Glandular tissues are replaced with fatty tissues.
    d. Parenchymal tissues become dense and opaque.

5. Which two projections comprise the standard examination for demonstrating the breasts?

    a. Craniocaudal and lateromedial
    b. Craniocaudal and mediolateral oblique
    c. Caudocranial and lateromedial
    d. Caudocranial and mediolateral oblique

6. Which projection requires that the central ray pass through the breast at an angle of 30 to 60 degrees?

    a. Axillary
    b. Caudocranial
    c. Craniocaudal
    d. Mediolateral oblique

7. Which muscle is often demonstrated with the craniocaudal projection?

    a. Pectoralis major
    b. Serratus anterior
    c. Rectus abdominis
    d. Lateral abdominal oblique

8. What is the primary objective of compressing the breast for mammography?

    a. To reduce exposure time
    b. To decrease geometric distortion
    c. To produce uniform breast thickness
    d. To produce uniform radiographic density

9. Where should the radiopaque marker, used to indicate which side is being examined, be seen on the image of craniocaudal projections?

    a. On the nipple
    b. On the chest wall
    c. Along the lateral side of the breast
    d. Along the medial side of the breast

10. How should a radiographer identify the location of a palpable mass?

    a. Draw a circle around the mass on the resultant mammogram.
    b. Use an ink marker to draw a circle on the skin overlying the mass.
    c. Place a radiopaque arrow marker alongside the breast to point to the mass.
    d. Place a radiopaque marker such as a BB on the breast overlying the mass.

11. What is the maximum difference for the length of the posterior nipple line when comparing images of craniocaudal and mediolateral oblique projections?

    a. 0.5 cm
    b. 1.0 cm
    c. 1.5 cm
    d. 2.0 cm

12. Between which two projections should the posterior nipple lines be measured and compared?

    a. Craniocaudal and mediolateral oblique
    b. Craniocaudal and 90-degree mediolateral
    c. Exaggerated craniocaudal and mediolateral oblique
    d. Exaggerated craniocaudal and 90-degree mediolateral

13. In which body position should the patient be placed for craniocaudal or mediolateral oblique projections?

    a. Prone
    b. Supine
    c. Upright
    d. Lateral recumbent

14. Which projection demonstrates all breast tissue with an emphasis on the lateral aspect and axillary tail?

    a. Mediolateral

    b. Craniocaudal

    c. Mediolateral oblique

    d. Exaggerated craniocaudal

15. Which projection requires that the central ray be moved to a horizontal position?

    a. Mediolateral

    b. Craniocaudal

    c. Mediolateral oblique

    d. Exaggerated craniocaudal

 If your school has access to Mosby's Radiographic Instructional Series on Anatomy, Positioning, and Procedures, review Unit 24 at this time. Your instructor may request that you respond to the series' exercises on paper. This unit covers the following topics of special interest:

Risk versus benefit

Breast imaging

Method of examination

The augmented breast

Localization of nonpalpable lesions for biopsy

Breast specimen radiography

Examination of milk ducts

CHAPTER 25

Central Nervous System

SECTION 1

Anatomy of the Central Nervous System

Instructions: This exercise pertains to the anatomic structures of the central nervous system (CNS). Identify structures, fill in missing words, or provide a short answer for each item.

1. Identify each lettered structure shown in Fig. 25-1.

   A. _____

   B. _____

   C. _____

   D. _____

   E. _____

   F. _____

   G. _____

   H. _____

2. Identify each lettered structure shown in Fig. 25-2.

   A. _____

   B. _____

   C. _____

   D. _____

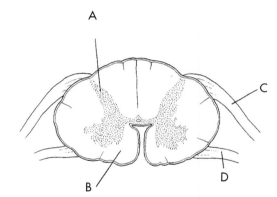

Fig. 25-2 Transverse section of the spinal cord.

Fig. 25-1 Lateral surface and midsection of the brain.

3. Identify each lettered structure shown in Fig. 25-3.

A. _____

B. _____

C. _____

D. _____

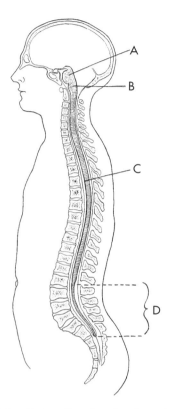

Fig. 25-3 Sagittal section showing the spinal cord.

4. Identify each lettered structure shown in Fig. 25-4.

A. _____

B. _____

C. _____

D. _____

E. _____

F. _____

G. _____

H. _____

Fig. 25-4 Lateral aspect of the cerebral ventricles in relation to the surface of the brain.

5. Identify each lettered structure shown in Fig. 25-5.

A. _____

B. _____

C. _____

Fig. 25-5 Anterior aspect of the lateral cerebral ventricles in relation to the surface of the brain.

6. Identify each lettered structure shown in Fig. 25-6.

A. _____

B. _____

C. _____

D. _____

E. _____

F. _____

G. _____

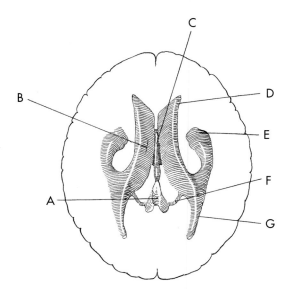

Fig. 25-6 Superior aspect of the cerebral ventricles in relation to the surface of the brain.

7. Name the two main parts of the central nervous system.

8. Name the three parts of the brain.

9. Name the four parts of the brain stem.

10. Name the three parts of the hindbrain.

11. The largest part of the brain is the

   _____.

12. Another name for the cerebrum is the

   _____.

13. The stemlike portion of the brain that connects the cere-

   brum to the hindbrain is the _____.

14. The deep cleft that separates the cerebrum into right and

   left hemispheres is the _____

   _____.

15. Another name for the hypophysis cerebri is

   _____ _____.

16. The largest part of the hindbrain is the

   _____.

17. The portion of the hindbrain that connects the pons to the

   spinal cord is the _____

   _____.

18. The protective membranes that enclose the brain and

   spinal cord are the _____.

19. The membrane that closely adheres to the brain and spinal

   cord is the _____

   _____.

20. The outermost membrane that forms the tough fibrous
   covering for the brain and spinal cord is the

   _____ _____.

21. The two uppermost ventricles are called the right and left

   _____ ventricles.

22. The lateral ventricles are located in the portion of the brain

   called the _____.

23. Each lateral ventricle communicates with the third ventri-

   cle by way of the _____ foramen.

24. Another name for the interventricular foramen is the fora-

   men of _____.

25. What are the two names for the passage between the third
   and fourth ventricles?

SECTION 2
Radiography of the Central Nervous System

Instructions: This exercise pertains to examinations that demonstrate central nervous system structures. Provide a short answer for each item.

1. Define myelography.

2. Identify three common sites for the injection of the contrast medium during myelography.

3. What abnormality is demonstrated using myelography?

4. What type or group of contrast media is preferred for myelography? Explain why.

5. When the exposure room is prepared for myelography, why should the spot-filming device be locked in place?

6. What should be done to reduce patient apprehension?

7. What are the two body positions most frequently used when the contrast medium is injected for myelography?

8. During myelography, what procedure is used to control the movement of the contrast medium after its injection?

9. During myelography, why should the patient hyperextend the neck?

10. When a traumatized patient with possible CNS involvement is radiographed, what radiograph should be the first one made?

Self-Test: Central Nervous System

Instructions: Answer the following questions by selecting the best choice.

1. Which two structures comprise the CNS?
   a. Brain and cerebellum
   b. Brain and spinal cord
   c. Cerebrum and cerebellum
   d. Cerebrum and spinal cord

2. Which part of the brain is also referred to as the forebrain?
   a. Pons
   b. Cerebrum
   c. Cerebellum
   d. Diencephalon

3. Which three parts of the CNS comprise the hindbrain?
   a. Cerebrum, cerebellum, and spinal cord
   b. Cerebrum, pons, and medulla oblongata
   c. Pons, cerebellum, and medulla oblongata
   d. Pons, spinal cord, and medulla oblongata

4. Which cerebral structure is the largest part of the brain?
   a. Pons
   b. Cerebrum
   c. Cerebellum
   d. Medulla oblongata

5. Which structure is divided into right and left hemispheres by the longitudinal fissure?
   a. Pons
   b. Cerebrum
   c. Cerebellum
   d. Medulla oblongata

6. What other term refers to the hypophysis cerebri?
   a. Pituitary gland
   b. Medulla spinalis
   c. Corpus callosum
   d. Conus medullaris

7. Which membrane forms the tough, fibrous outer covering for the meninges?
   a. Pia mater
   b. Arachnoid
   c. Dura mater

8. Which vessel connects the lateral ventricles to the third ventricle?
   a. Cerebral aqueduct
   b. Foramen of Luschka
   c. Foramen of Magendie
   d. Interventricular foramen

9. In which part of the brain is the fourth ventricle found?
   a. Midbrain
   b. Forebrain
   c. Hindbrain

10. Which projection should be the first radiograph for a traumatized patient with possible CNS involvement?
    a. AP axial
    b. AP oblique
    c. Upright lateral
    d. Cross-table lateral

11. Which examination is performed to demonstrate the contour of the subarachnoid space?
    a. Diskography
    b. Myelography
    c. Ventriculography
    d. Pneumonography

12. For which examination is the contrast medium injected directly into the fibrous cartilage between two vertebral bodies?
    a. Diskography
    b. Myelography
    c. Ventriculography
    d. Pneumonography

13. Which examination can be used to evaluate the dynamic flow pattern of cerebral spinal fluid?
    a. Diskography
    b. Myelography
    c. Ventriculography
    d. Pneumonography

14. During myelography, which procedure should be performed to prevent contrast medium from entering the cerebral ventricles?
    a. Tilt the head of the table down.
    b. Instruct the patient to hyperflex the neck.
    c. Place the patient in the lateral recumbent position.
    d. Have the patient hyperextend the neck

15. What is the purpose of tilting the table during myelography?
    a. To attach the footboard
    b. To facilitate patient comfort
    c. To control the flow of contrast medium
    d. To remove cerebral spinal fluid from the patient

If your school has access to Mosby's Radiographic Instructional Series on Anatomy, Positioning, and Procedures, review Unit 25 at this time. Your instructor may request that you respond to the series' exercises on paper. This unit covers the following examinations:

Plain radiographic examination
Myelography
   Contrast media
   Computed tomography
Diskography
Chemonucleolysis
Magnetic resonance imaging
Cerebral pneumonography/ventriculography
Stereotactic surgery

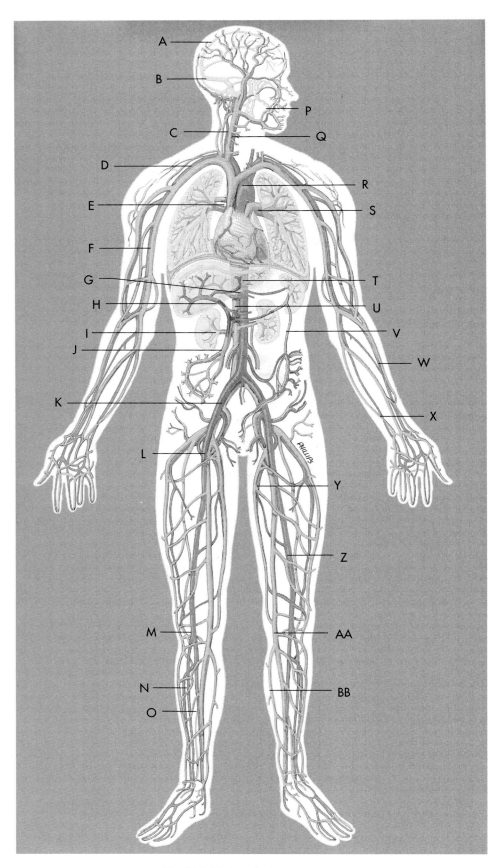

Fig. 26-1 Major arteries and veins.

CHAPTER 26

Circulatory System

SECTION 1

Anatomy of the Circulatory System

Exercise 1

Instructions: This exercise pertains to the anatomy of the circulatory system. Identify structures for each item.

1. Identify each lettered structure shown in Fig. 26-1 (see opposite page).

A. _____

B. _____

C. _____

D. _____

E. _____

F. _____

G. _____

H. _____

I. _____

J. _____

K. _____

L. _____

M. _____

N. _____

O. _____

P. _____

Q. _____

R. _____

S. _____

T. _____

U. _____

V. _____

W. _____

X. _____

Y. _____

Z. _____

AA. _____

BB. _____

2. Identify each lettered structure shown in Fig. 26-2.

A. _____

B. _____

C. _____

D. _____

E. _____

F. _____

G. _____

H. _____

I. _____

J. _____

K. _____

L. _____

M. _____

3. Identify each lettered structure shown in Fig. 26-3.

A. _____

B. _____

Fig. 26-3 Anterior view of the coronary arteries.

4. Identify each lettered structure shown in Fig. 26-4.

A. _____

B. _____

Fig. 26-2 The heart and greater vessels. *Black arrows* indicate deoxygenated blood flow. *White arrows* indicate oxygenated blood flow.

Fig. 26-4 Anterior view of the coronary veins.

5. Identify each lettered structure shown in Fig. 26-5.

A. _____

B. _____

C. _____

D. _____

E. _____

F. _____

G. _____

H. _____

I. _____

J. _____

K. _____

L. _____

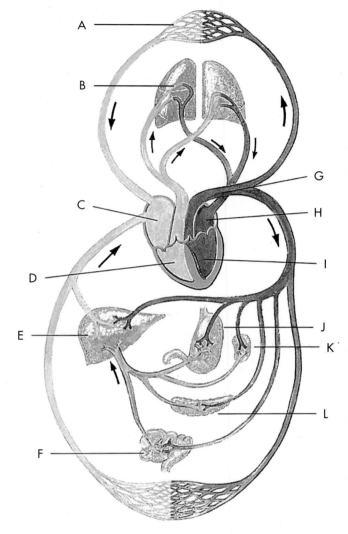

Fig. 26-5 The pulmonary, systemic, and portal circulation.

6. Identify each lettered structure shown in Fig. 26-6.

A. _____   H. _____

B. _____   I. _____

C. _____   J. _____

D. _____   K. _____

E. _____   L. _____

F. _____   M. _____

G. _____

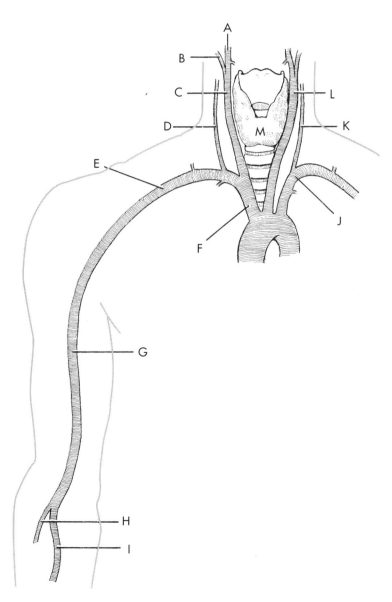

Fig. 26-6 Major arteries of the upper chest, neck, and arm.

7. Identify each lettered structure shown in Fig. 26-7.

A. _____

B. _____

C. _____

D. _____

E. _____

F. _____

G. _____

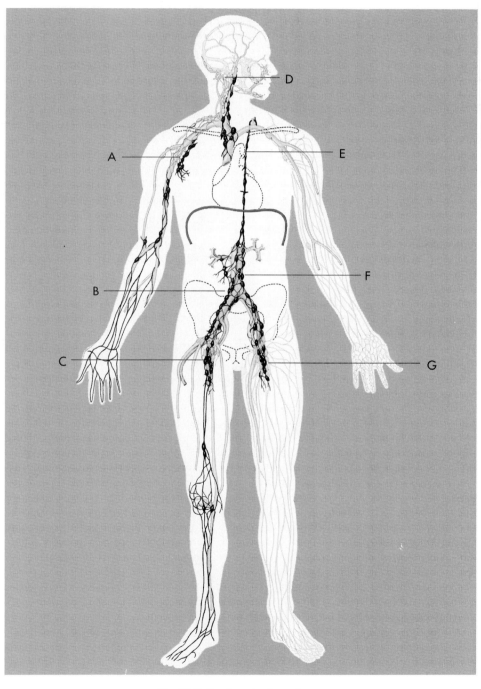

Fig. 26-7 The lymphatic system.

Exercise 2

Instructions: This exercise is a comprehensive review of the circulatory system. Fill in missing words for each item.

1. The circulatory system comprises two systems of related vessels, the _____ system and the _____ system.

2. The two systems that comprise the blood-vascular system are _____ circulation and _____ circulation.

3. The system that traverses the lungs to discharge carbon dioxide and take up oxygen is _____ circulation.

4. The vessels that carry blood away from the heart are collectively called _____.

5. The vessels that carry blood back toward the heart are collectively called _____.

6. Arteries subdivide to form _____.

7. Arterioles subdivide to form _____.

8. Capillaries unite to form _____.

9. The beginning branches for veins are _____.

10. Blood is transported to the left atrium by _____ veins.

11. The major vein that returns blood from the upper parts of the body to the heart is the _____ _____ _____.

12. The major vein that returns blood from the lower parts of the body to the heart is the _____ _____ _____.

13. The muscular wall of the heart is the _____.

14. The membrane that lines the chambers of the heart is the _____.

15. The membrane that covers the heart is the _____.

16. The chamber of the heart where the myocardium is the thickest is the _____ _____.

17. The space between the two walls of the pericardial sac is the _____ _____.

18. The two upper chambers of the heart are the _____.

19. The two lower chambers of the heart are the _____.

20. The receiving chambers of the heart are the _____.

21. The distributing chambers of the heart are the _____.

22. Another name for the right atrioventricular valve is the _____ valve.

23. Two other terms that refer to the left atrioventricular valve are the _____ valve and the _____ valve.

24. The side of the heart that pumps venous (deoxygenated) blood is the _____ (right or left) side.

25. The side of the heart that pumps arterial (oxygenated) blood is the _____ (right or left) side.

26. The chamber of the heart that pumps blood through the aortic valve is the _____ _____.

27. The vessels that supply blood to the myocardium are the right and left _____ arteries.

28. The coronary sinus receives blood from the _____ veins.

29. The coronary sinus empties blood into the _____ (right or left) atrium.

30. The great vessel that arises from the left ventricle to transport blood to the body is the _____.

31. The abdominal aorta divides into the right and left common _____ arteries.

32. The external iliac artery enters the lower limb and becomes the _____ artery.

33. The femoral artery passes blood into the _____ artery.

34. The popliteal artery bifurcates into the anterior and posterior _____ arteries.

35. The vessel that drains blood into the liver is the _____ vein.

36. The vessels that drain blood from the liver are the _____ veins.

37. Hepatic veins transport blood to the _____ _____ _____.

38. The large vessel that arises from the right atrium is the _____ artery.

39. The only arteries of the body that transport deoxygenated blood are the _____ arteries.

40. The only veins of the body that transport oxygenated blood are the _____ veins.

41. The contraction phase of the heart is called the _____.

42. The relaxation phase of the heart is called the _____.

43. The four arteries that supply the brain are the right and left _____ _____ arteries and the right and left _____ arteries.

44. Of the four trunk arteries that supply the brain, the one that arises directly from the arch of the aorta is the _____ _____ _____ artery.

45. The right and left vertebral arteries arise from the _____ arteries.

46. The right and left vertebral arteries unite to form the _____ artery.

47. Each common carotid artery bifurcates into the _____ and _____ carotid arteries.

48. Each internal carotid artery bifurcates into anterior and middle _____ arteries.

49. The basilar artery bifurcates into the right and left _____ _____ arteries.

50. Blood is drained from the head by the

    _____ veins.

51. To reach the right subclavian artery, blood passes from the

    aorta through the _____ artery.

52. Blood passes from the brachiocephalic artery to the right

    _____ artery.

53. A subclavian artery supplies blood to the axillary artery

    and then to the _____ artery.

54. The brachial arteries bifurcate into the

    _____ and

    _____ arteries.

55. The part of the body in which the cephalic vein originates

    is the _____.

56. The renal arteries arise from the

    _____.

57. The circle of Willis is located within the

    _____.

58. The central organ of the blood-vascular system is the

    _____.

59. The main terminal trunk of the lymphatic system is the

    _____ duct.

60. The thoracic duct drains its contents at the junction of the

    left _____ vein and the internal

    _____ vein.

SECTION 2

Radiography of the Circulatory System

Instructions: This exercise pertains to various radiographic examinations for the circulatory system. Because many of these procedures are dependent upon the preferences of the radiologist, most of the following exercise items are general in content rather than emphasizing a specific procedure. Identify structures, fill in missing words, select from a list, or provide a short answer for each item.

1. List four reasons that catheterization is preferred over direct injection of the contrast medium through a needle.

2. The most widely used method of catheterization is the

   _____ technique.

3. The preferred site for insertion of the catheter for most

   selective angiography is the _____
   artery.

4. What is the purpose of side holes near the tip of the catheter?

   a. To draw fluid into the catheter
   b. To reduce whiplash, stabilizing the catheter
   c. To maintain positive pressure inside the catheter

5. From the list below, circle the three symptoms of a vasovagal reaction that are caused by the injection of the contrast medium.

   a. Hives
   b. Nausea
   c. Sweating
   d. Difficult breathing
   e. Increase in pulse rate
   f. Increase in blood pressure
   g. Decrease in blood pressure

6. From the list below, circle the three symptoms of shock.

   a. Low pulse rate
   b. High pulse rate
   c Rapid breathing
   d. Shallow breathing
   e. Loss of consciousness
   f. Rise in body temperature

7. What treatment should be given to patients experiencing low blood pressure because of a vasovagal reaction?

8. In preparation for angiography, why should the patient be instructed not to consume solid food?

9. In preparation for angiography, why should the patient be allowed to drink clear liquids?

10. For thoracic aortography, to which vertebra should the perpendicular central ray be directed?

    _____

11. Identify each lettered structure shown in Fig. 26-8.

A. _____   E. _____

B. _____   F. _____

C. _____   G. _____

D. _____   H. _____

Fig. 26-8 AP thoracic aortogram.

12. How much of the aorta should be imaged for abdominal aortography?

13. For abdominal aortography, which projection of the abdominal aorta—AP or lateral—best demonstrates the celiac and superior mesenteric artery origins?

   _____

14. Identify each lettered structure shown in Fig. 26-9.

   A. _____

   B. _____

   C. _____

   D. _____

   E. _____

   F. _____

Fig. 26-9 AP abdominal aortogram.

15. Identify each lettered structure shown in Fig. 26-10.

   A. _____

   B. _____

   C. _____

Fig. 26-10 Lateral abdominal aortogram.

16. For pulmonary arteriography, which projection—AP or lateral—should use a compensating (trough) filter to obtain a radiograph with more uniform density between the vertebrae and the lungs?

   _____

17. All radiographs for selective abdominal visceral arteriography should be exposed when the patient has suspended

   _____ (inspiration or expiration).

Fig. 26-11 Selective AP celiac arteriogram.

18. Identify each lettered structure shown in Fig. 26-11.

A. _____

B. _____

C. _____

D. _____

E. _____

19. What is the advantage of examining the patient's intravenous urography radiographs before positioning the patient for a renal arteriogram?

20. For demonstrating the portal venous system, the contrast medium should be injected into the

_____ artery.

21. Blood in veins flows _____ (proximally or distally).

22. For renal venography, the renal vein is most easily catheterized using the _____ (upper or lower) limb approach.

23. Into which vein should a catheter be positioned to best demonstrate the superior vena cava?

a. Subclavian
b. Common iliac
c. Inferior vena cava

24. Into which vein should a catheter be positioned to best demonstrate the inferior vena cava?

a. Portal
b. Common iliac
c. Superior vena cava

25. Into which artery should the catheter be positioned to best demonstrate the arteries of an entire upper limb with a single injection of contrast medium?

a. Femoral
b. Subclavian
c. Common iliac

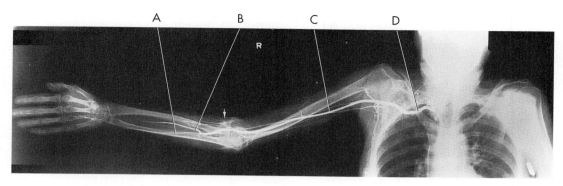

Fig. 26-12 Right upper-limb arteriogram. (The radial artery is not demonstrated due to occlusion.)

26. Identify each lettered structure shown in Fig. 26-12.

    A. _____

    B. _____

    C. _____

    D. _____

27. Where is the injection site for the introduction of contrast medium for upper limb venography?

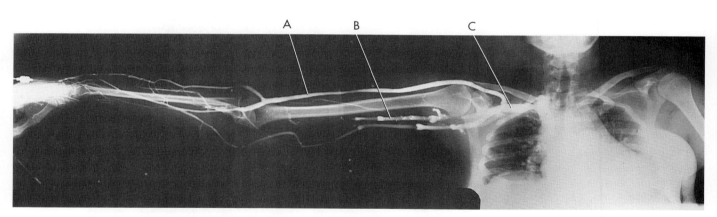

Fig. 26-13 Right upper-limb venogram.

28. Identify each lettered structure shown in Fig. 26-13.

    A. _____

    B. _____

    C. _____

29. For simultaneous bilateral femoral arteriograms, how should the patient's legs be positioned?

30. Identify each lettered structure shown in Fig. 26-14.

A. _____

B. _____

C. _____

D. _____

E. _____

F. _____

G. _____

H. _____

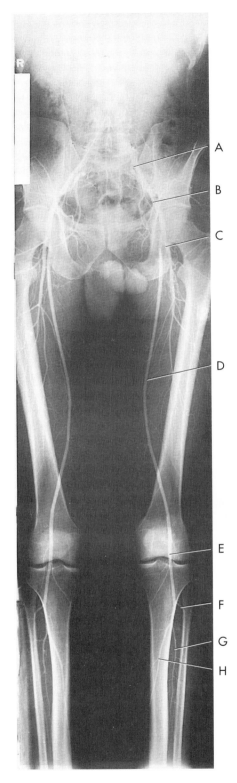

Fig. 26-14 Normal aortofemoral arteriogram in the late arterial phase.

31. At what area of the leg should radiographs begin for lower limb venography?

    a. Hip

    b. Knee

    c. Ankle

32. For lower limb venography, what is the purpose of applying tourniquets just proximal to the ankle and knee?

    a. To stop the pulse within the leg

    b. To prevent blood flow into the leg

    c. To force the filling of the deep veins of the leg

33. Approximately how many seconds does it take for blood to flow from the internal carotid artery to the jugular vein in cerebral angiography?

    a. 3 seconds

    b. 6 seconds

    c. 9 seconds

34. Why should the first radiograph of a cerebral arteriography series be made before the arrival of the contrast medium?

    a. To check exposure factors

    b. To confirm patient positioning

    c. To serve as a subtraction mask

    d. To demonstrate soft tissue abnormalities

35. What is the visualization sequence for the three phases of blood flow that should be seen in cerebral angiography?

    a. Arterial, capillary, and venous

    b. Arterial, venous, and capillary

    c. Capillary, arterial, and venous

    d. Capillary, venous, and arterial

    e. Venous, arterial, and capillary

    f. Venous, capillary, and arterial

Fig. 26-15 Cerebral angiogram.

Fig. 26-16 Cerebral angiogram.

Fig. 26-17 Cerebral angiogram.

36. Figs. 26-15, 26-16, and 26-17 are cerebral angiograms, and each shows a phase of blood flow. Examine each image and identify which phase of blood flow—arterial, capillary, or venous—the image represents.

a. Figure 26-15: _____

b. Figure 26-16: _____

c. Figure 26-17: _____

37. For the basic AP projection during cerebral angiography, what positioning line of the skull should be perpendicular to the horizontal plane?

_____

38. For the AP axial oblique projection (transorbital) demonstrating anterior circulation during cerebral angiography, in which direction—toward the injected side or away from the injected side—should the head be rotated?

39. For the AP axial projection (supraorbital) demonstrating anterior circulation during cerebral angiography, how should the central ray be directed to project the vessels above the floor of the anterior cranial fossa?
   a. Caudally
   b. Cephalically
   c. Perpendicularly

40. For the AP axial oblique projection (transorbital) demonstrating the internal carotid bifurcation and the anterior communicating and middle cerebral arteries within the orbital shadow, how should the central ray be directed?
   a. Caudally
   b. Cephalically
   c. Perpendicularly

Self-Test: Anatomy and Radiography of the Circulatory System

Instructions: Answer the following questions by selecting the best choice.

1. Which vessels originate immediately because of the division of arteries?

   a. Veins
   b. Venules
   c. Arterioles
   d. Capillaries

2. In which part of the body is the basilic vein located?

   a. Head
   b. Abdomen
   c. Lower limb
   d. Upper limb

3. Which chamber of the heart receives deoxygenated blood?

   a. Left atrium
   b. Left ventricle
   c. Right atrium
   d. Right ventricle

4. Which chamber of the heart receives blood from the pulmonary veins?

   a. Left atrium
   b. Left ventricle
   c. Right atrium
   d. Right ventricle

5. What is the purpose of the septa of the heart?

   a. To separate atria from ventricles
   b. To provide openings into the atria
   c. To form the atrioventricular valves
   d. To divide the heart into right and left halves

6. The circuit for blood flow from the left ventricle to the right atrium is the _____ circulation.

   a. Deep
   b. Systemic
   c. Superficial
   d. Pulmonary

7. Which arteries are the first to branch from the ascending aorta?

   a. Coronary
   b. Vertebral
   c. Subclavian
   d. Common carotid

8. Through which valve does blood pass when it exits the heart for systemic circulation?

   a. Aortic
   b. Mitral
   c. Bicuspid
   d. Tricuspid

9. Which of the following is a disadvantage of nonionic contrast agents compared with ionic contrast agents of lower iodine concentrations?

   a. Increased viscosity
   b. Increased cardiovascular side effects
   c. Increased exposure factor requirements
   d. Decreased radiographic contrast of opacified vessels

10. Why can exposures not occur in both planes at the same moment during simultaneous biplane imaging?

    a. X-ray tubes will overload.
    b. Scatter radiation will fog the images.
    c. Two injections of contrast medium are required.
    d. X-ray generators cannot be synchronized for multiple exposures.

11. Which procedure should be performed to reduce the magnification of structures for lateral projections during thoracic aortography?

    a. Use a cassette changer.
    b. Use the smallest available focal spot.
    c. Increase the source-to-image receptor distance (SID).
    d. Increase the object-to-image receptor distance (OID).

12. Which arteriogram requires the use of a compensating (trough) filter to obtain a more uniform density between the vertebral structures and lungs?

    a. AP celiac axis
    b. AP pulmonary
    c. Lateral pulmonary
    d. AP superior mesenteric

13. To which level of the patient should the cassette and central ray be centered for AP abdominal aortograms?

    a. T6
    b. T10
    c. L2
    d. Iliac crests

14. To which level of the patient should the cassette and central ray be centered for celiac arteriograms?

    a. T2
    b. T6
    c. L2
    d. S1

15. Which area of the patient should be prepared for the injection of contrast medium for cephalic venography?

    a. Thigh
    b. Ankle
    c. Wrist
    d. Upper arm

16. Which area of the patient should be prepared for the injection of contrast medium for demonstration of the superior vena cava?

    a. Thigh
    b. Ankle
    c. Wrist
    d. Upper arm

17. Which area of the patient is the preferred site for insertion of the catheter through the skin for internal carotid arteriography?

    a. Neck
    b. Thigh
    c. Abdomen
    d. Upper arm

18. Why should a radiograph be taken before the arrival of contrast medium for cerebral angiography?

    a. To serve as a subtraction mask
    b. To ensure that collimation is adequate
    c. To check for proper positioning of the patient
    d. To verify that the correct exposure factors are used

19. Which phase of blood flow should have the most films exposed during cerebral angiography?

    a. Venous
    b. Arterial
    c. Capillary
    d. Parenchymal

20. Which positioning line of the skull should be perpendicular to the horizontal plane for basic AP projections during cerebral arteriography?

    a. Orbitomeatal
    b. Glabellomeatal
    c. Acanthiomeatal
    d. Infraorbitomeatal

If your school has access to Mosby's Radiographic Instructional Series on Anatomy, Positioning, and Procedures, review Unit 26 at this time. Your instructor may request that you respond to the series' exercises on paper. This unit covers selected aspects of the following examinations:

Diagnostic visceral and peripheral angiography
Cerebral angiography
Interventional radiology
Lymphography
Photographic subtraction technique

CHAPTER 27

Sectional Anatomy for Radiographers

Review

Instructions: An understanding of the relationships between organ and skeletal structures by the radiographer is essential in computed tomography (CT), magnetic resonance imaging (MRI), and diagnostic ultrasound examinations because all three modalities create images of sectional anatomy. This exercise is a review of sectional anatomy. Identify structures for each item.

Fig. 27-1 shows a CT localizer, or scout, image of the skull. Figs. 27-2 through 27-5 pertain to the imaging planes shown in Fig. 27-1.

1. Identify each lettered structure shown in Fig. 27-2.

   A. _____

   B. _____

   C. _____

   D. _____

   E. _____

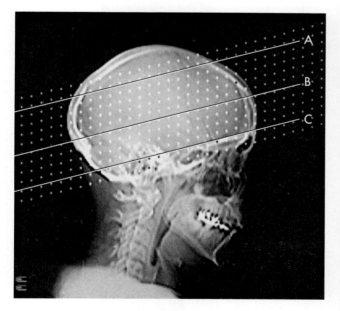

Fig. 27-1 CT localizer, or scout, image of the skull.

Fig. 27-2 CT image corresponding to level *A* in Fig. 27-1.

2. Identify each lettered structure shown in Fig. 27-3.

A. _____   F. _____

B. _____   G. _____

C. _____   H. _____

D. _____   I. _____

E. _____   J. _____

Fig. 27-3 MRI image corresponding to level *B* in Fig. 27-1.

3. Identify each lettered structure shown in Fig. 27-4.

A. _____ G. _____

B. _____ H. _____

C. _____ I. _____

D. _____ J. _____

E. _____ K. _____

F. _____

Fig. 27-4 CT image corresponding to level *C* in Fig. 27-1.

4. Identify each lettered structure shown in Fig. 27-5.

A. _____

B. _____

C. _____

D. _____

E. _____

F. _____

G. _____

H. _____

I. _____

J. _____

K. _____

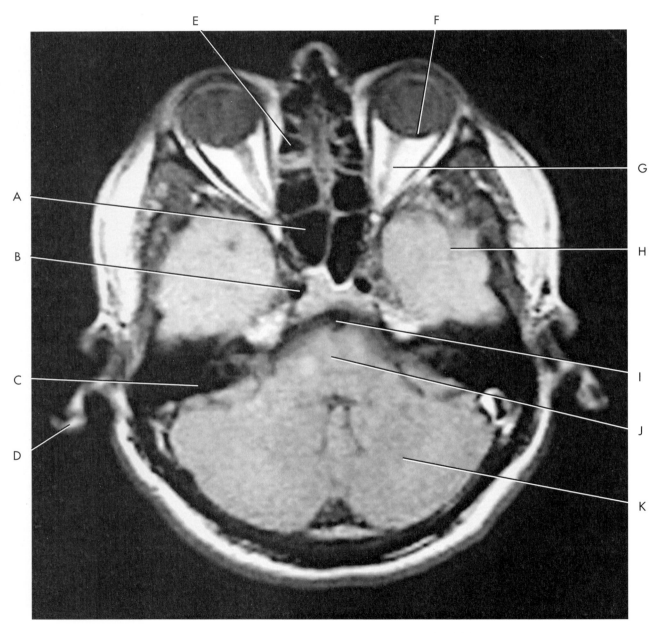

Fig. 27-5 MRI image corresponding to level *C* in Fig. 27-1.

5. Identify each lettered structure shown in Fig. 27-6.

A. _____

B. _____

C. _____

D. _____

E. _____

F. _____

G. _____

H. _____

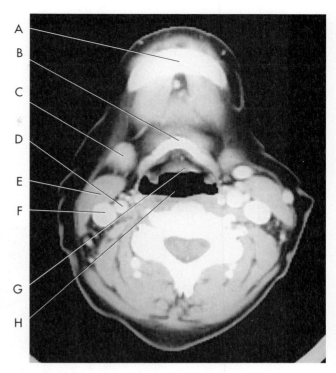

Fig. 27-6 CT image through the fourth cervical vertebra.

6. Identify each lettered structure shown in Fig. 27-7.

A. _____

B. _____

C. _____

D. _____

E. _____

F. _____

G. _____

H. _____

I. _____

Fig. 27-7 CT image through the sixth cervical vertebra.

7. Identify each lettered structure shown in Fig. 27-8.

A. _____

B. _____

C. _____

D. _____

E. _____

F. _____

G. _____

H. _____

I. _____

J. _____

K. _____

L. _____

M. _____

N. _____

O. _____

P. _____

Q. _____

R. _____

S. _____

T. _____

Fig. 27-8 Sagittal MRI image through the medial sagittal plane.

Fig. 27-9 shows a CT localizer, or scout, image of the skull. Figs. 27-10, 27-11, and 27-12 pertain to the imaging planes shown in Fig. 27-9.

Fig. 27-9 CT localizer, or scout, image of the skull.

8. Identify each lettered structure shown in Fig. 27-10.

A. _____

B. _____

C. _____

D. _____

E. _____

F. _____

G. _____

H. _____

I. _____

J. _____

K. _____

L. _____

M. _____

N. _____

O. _____

P. _____

Q. _____

R. _____

S. _____

Fig. 27-10 Coronal MRI image corresponding to level *A* in Fig. 27-9.

9. Identify each lettered structure shown in Fig. 27-11.

A. _____   G. _____

B. _____   H. _____

C. _____   I. _____

D. _____   J. _____

E. _____   K. _____

F. _____

Fig. 27-11 Coronal MRI image corresponding to level *B* in Fig. 27-9.

10. Identify each lettered structure shown in Fig. 27-12.

A. _____

B. _____

C. _____

D. _____

E. _____

F. _____

G. _____

H. _____

I. _____

J. _____

K. _____

Fig. 27-12 Coronal MRI image corresponding to level *C* in Fig. 27-9.

Fig. 27-13 shows a CT localizer, or scout, image of the thorax. Figs. 27-14, 27-15, and 27-16 pertain to the imaging planes shown in Fig. 27-13.

Fig. 27-13 CT localizer, or scout, image of the thorax.

11. Identify each lettered structure shown in Fig. 27-14.

A. _____

B. _____

C. _____

D. _____

E. _____

F. _____

G. _____

H. _____

I. _____

J. _____

12. Identify each lettered structure shown in Fig. 27-15.

A. _____

B. _____

C. _____

D. _____

E. _____

F. _____

G. _____

H. _____

I. _____

J. _____

K. _____

Fig. 27-14 CT image corresponding to level *A* at the second thoracic vertebra in Fig. 27-13.

Fig. 27-15 CT image corresponding to level *B* at the fifth thoracic vertebra in Fig. 27-13.

13. Identify each lettered structure shown in Fig. 27-16.

A. _____

B. _____

C. _____

D. _____

E. _____

F. _____

G. _____

H. _____

I. _____

J. _____

K. _____

Fig. 27-16 CT image corresponding to level *C* at the ninth thoracic vertebra in Fig. 27-13.

14. Identify each lettered structure shown in Fig. 27-17.

A. _____

B. _____

C. _____

D. _____

E. _____

F. _____

G. _____

H. _____

I. _____

J. _____

K. _____

L. _____

Fig. 27-17 Median sagittal MRI image through the neck and upper thorax.

15. Identify each lettered structure shown in Fig. 27-18.

A. _____

B. _____

C. _____

D. _____

E. _____

F. _____

G. _____

H. _____

I. _____

J. _____

K. _____

Fig. 27-18 MRI image of the neck and thorax through the median coronal plane.

Fig. 27-19 shows a CT localizer, or scout, image of the abdominopelvic region. Figs. 27-20 through 27-26 pertain to the imaging planes shown in Fig. 27-19.

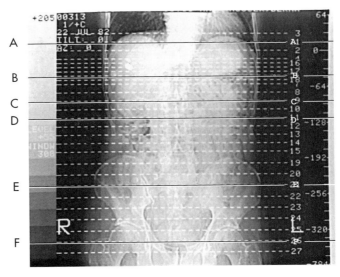

Fig. 27-19 CT localizer, or scout, image of the abdominopelvic region.

16. Identify each lettered structure shown in Fig. 27-20.

A. _____

B. _____

C. _____

D. _____

E. _____

F. _____

G. _____

Fig. 27-20 CT image corresponding to level *A* at the tenth thoracic vertebra in Fig. 27-19.

17. Identify each lettered structure shown in Fig. 27-21.

A. _____

B. _____

C. _____

D. _____

E. _____

F. _____

G. _____

H. _____

I. _____

J. _____

K. _____

Fig. 27-21 CT image corresponding to level *B* at the twelfth thoracic vertebra in Fig. 27-19.

18. Identify each lettered structure shown in Fig. 27-22.

A. _____

B. _____

C. _____

D. _____

E. _____

F. _____

G. _____

H. _____

I. _____

J. _____

Fig. 27-22 CT image corresponding to level *C* at the second lumbar vertebra in Fig. 27-19.

19. Identify each lettered structure shown in Fig. 27-23.

A. _____   E. _____

B. _____   F. _____

C. _____   G. _____

D. _____

Fig. 27-23 CT image corresponding to level *D* at the interspace between the second and third lumbar vertebrae in Fig. 27-19.

20. Identify each lettered structure shown in Fig. 27-24.

A. _____   E. _____

B. _____   F. _____

C. _____   G. _____

D. _____

Fig. 27-24 CT image corresponding to level *E* at the anterior superior ilias spine (ASIS) in Fig. 27-19.

21. Identify each lettered structure shown in Fig. 27-25.

A. _____

B. _____

C. _____

D. _____

E. _____

F. _____

G. _____

Fig. 27-25 CT image corresponding to level *F* at the coccyx (female) in Fig. 27-19.

22. Identify each lettered structure shown in Fig. 27-26.

A. _____   G. _____

B. _____   H. _____

C. _____   I. _____

D. _____   J. _____

E. _____   K. _____

F. _____   L. _____

Fig. 27-26 CT image corresponding to level *F* at the coccyx (male) in Fig. 27-19.

23. Identify each lettered structure shown in Fig. 27-27.

A. _____

B. _____

C. _____

D. _____

E. _____

F. _____

G. _____

H. _____

I. _____

J. _____

K. _____

L. _____

M. _____

Fig. 27-27 MRI image of the abdominopelvic region at the median sagittal plane.

24. Identify each lettered structure shown in Fig. 27-28.

A. _____

B. _____

C. _____

D. _____

E. _____

F. _____

G. _____

H. _____

I. _____

J. _____

K. _____

L. _____

M. _____

N. _____

Fig. 27-28 MRI image of the abdominopelvic region at the median coronal plane.

If your school has access to Mosby's Radiographic Instructional Series on Anatomy, Positioning, and Procedures, review Unit 27 at this time. Your instructor may request that you respond to the series' exercises on paper. This unit covers the examination techniques for the following anatomic regions:

Cranial region
Thoracic region
Abdominopelvic region

Supplemental Exercises for Skull Positioning

Skull Positioning Review

Note to Students: The exercises in this appendix pertain to information referenced from Chapters 20 through 23 and should be completed *after* you have completed the review exercises for those four chapters.

Exercise 1

Instructions: Match each projection in Column A with the number of degrees and direction of central ray angulation in Column B. Choices from Column B may be used once, more than once, or not at all.

Column A

_____ 1. AP axial (facial bones)

_____ 2. AP axial (cranium, Towne method)

_____ 3. AP axial (temporomandibular articulations)

_____ 4. AP axial (zygomatic arches, modified Towne method)

_____ 5. PA (sphenoidal sinuses)

_____ 6. PA axial (cranium, Haas method)

_____ 7. PA axial (sinuses, Caldwell method)

_____ 8. PA axial (cranium, Caldwell method)

_____ 9. Axiolateral oblique (mandible)

_____ 10. Axiolateral oblique (temporomandibular articulations)

_____ 11. Axiolateral oblique (petromastoid portion, Arcelin method [anterior profile])

_____ 12. Axiolateral oblique (petromastoid portion, Stenvers method [posterior profile])

_____ 13. Parietoacanthial (sinuses, Waters method)

_____ 14. Parieto-orbital oblique (optic foramen, Rhese method)

_____ 15. Axiolateral (mastoids, modified Law method [single-tube angulation method])

Column B

a. Perpendicular

b. 10 degrees caudad

c. 10 degrees cephalad

d. 12 degrees caudad

e. 12 degrees cephalad

f. 15 degrees caudad

g. 15 degrees cephalad

h. 20 degrees caudad

i. 20 degrees cephalad

j. 23 degrees caudad

k. 23 degrees cephalad

l. 25 degrees caudad

m. 25 degrees cephalad

n. 30 degrees caudad

o. 30 degrees cephalad

p. 35 degrees caudad

q. 35 degrees cephalad

r. 37 degrees cephalad

Exercise 2

Instructions: Match the projections in Column A with the locations in Column B. Each location in Column B is either a centering point for the body part or a point where the central ray should enter or exit the patient. Not all locations in Column B may apply to the projections listed in Column B.

Column A

_____ 1. Lateral (cranium)

_____ 2. Lateral (nasal bones)

_____ 3. Lateral (facial bones)

_____ 4. Lateral (sella turcica)

_____ 5. Lateral (paranasal sinuses)

_____ 6. Tangential (zygomatic arch)

_____ 7. PA axial (cranium, Haas method)

_____ 8. PA axial (cranium, Caldwell method)

_____ 9. Parietoacanthial (sinuses, Waters method)

_____ 10. AP axial (zygomatic arches)

_____ 11. AP axial (temporomandibular articulations)

_____ 12. Axiolateral oblique (temporomandibular articulations)

_____ 13. Axiolateral oblique (petromastoid portion, Arcelin method [anterior profile])

_____ 14. Axiolateral oblique (petromastoid portion, Stenvers method [posterior profile])

_____ 15. Axiolateral (mastoids, modified Law method [single-tube angulation method])

Column B

a. Nasion

b. Glabella

c. Acanthion

d. Zygomatic bone

e. External acoustic meatus

f. ½ inch (1.2 cm) distal to the nasion

g. 1½ inches (4 cm) above the nasion

h. 3 inches (7.5 cm) above the nasion

i. ½ to 1 inch (1.2 to 2.5 cm) posterior to the outer canthus

j. 1½ inches (4 cm) posterior to the outer canthus

k. ½ inch (1.2 cm) anterior to the external acoustic meatus

l. 1 inch (2.5 cm) anterior to the external acoustic meatus

m. 1 inch (2.5 cm) posterior to the external acoustic meatus

n. 2 inches (5 cm) superior to the external acoustic meatus

o. ¾ inch (2 cm) anterior and ¾ inch (2 cm) superior to the external acoustic meatus

p. 1 inch (2.5 cm) anterior and ¾ inch (2 cm) superior to the external acoustic meatus

Exercise 3

Instructions: Examine the following diagrams of various projections of the skull (e.g., cranium, facial bones, sinuses). Listed after the diagrams are the names and characteristics of skull projections. In the space provided, write the letter of the diagram that corresponds to each name or characteristic. Not all diagrams may apply to the listed names and characteristics, and some diagrams may be used more than once.

F

G

H

I

J

K

L

M

N

O

P

Q

R

S

_____ 1. Parietoacanthial projection (Waters method)

_____ 2. Full basal projection of the cranium

_____ 3. AP axial projection (cranium, Towne method)

_____ 4. AP axial projection demonstrating facial bones

_____ 5. PA axial projection (cranium, Haas method)

_____ 6. PA axial projection (cranium, Caldwell method)

_____ 7. PA projection to demonstrate sphenoidal sinuses

_____ 8. Orbitoparietal oblique projection (Rhese method)

_____ 9. Parietoorbital oblique projection (Rhese method)

_____ 10. Demonstrates one temporomandibular joint

_____ 11. Best projection for demonstrating the maxillary sinuses

_____ 12. Tangential projection for demonstrating an individual zygomatic arch

_____ 13. Petrous ridges should be projected immediately below the maxillae

_____ 14. Demonstrates the mastoid air cells of the side closest to the cassette

_____ 15. Lateral projection and central ray alignment for demonstrating the nasal bones

_____ 16. Lateral projection and central ray alignment for demonstrating the facial bones

_____ 17. Orbitomeatal line should form an angle of 37 degrees with the cassette

_____ 18. Petrous ridges should be projected into the lower one third of the orbits

_____ 19. Shows a profile image of the part of the petromastoid closest to the cassette

_____ 20. Axiolateral oblique projection (petromastoid portion, Arcelin method [anterior profile])

_____ 21. Axiolateral oblique projection (petromastoid portion, Stenvers method [posterior profile])

_____ 22. AP axial projection and central ray alignment for demonstrating bilateral zygomatic arches

_____ 23. AP axial projection and central ray alignment for demonstrating temporomandibular joints

_____ 24. Produces a slightly oblique tangential image of one zygomatic arch free from superimposed shadows

_____ 25. Central ray should enter 2 inches (5 cm) posterior to and 2 inches (5 cm) superior to the upside external acoustic meatus

Answers to Exercises

CHAPTER 14 **Mouth and Salivary Glands**

Review

1. A. Posterior arch
   B. Anterior arch
   C. Tonsil
   D. Hard palate
   E. Uvula
   F. Soft palate
   G. Tongue
2. A. Orifice of the submandibular duct
   B. Tongue
   C. Frenulum of the tongue
   D. Sublingual fold
3. A. Parotid duct
   B. Sublingual ducts
   C. Submandibular duct
   D. Sublingual gland
   E. Parotid gland
   F. Submandibular gland
4. A. Muscle tissue
   B. Ramus of mandible
   C. Parotid gland
   D. Tongue
   E. Dens
   F. Atlas
   G. Spinal cord
5. A. Mandible
   B. Oropharynx
   C. Cervical vertebral body
   D. Sublingual gland
   E. Submandibular gland
   F. Tip of parotid gland
6. Mouth
7. The process of chewing and grinding food into small pieces
8. Teeth
9. To soften food, keep the mouth moist, and contribute digestive enzymes
10. Parotid, sublingual, and submandibular
11. Radiographic examination of the salivary glands and ducts with the use of a contrast medium
12. Water-soluble, iodinated medium
13. Salivary gland pairs are in close proximity.
14. To detect any condition demonstrable without the use of a contrast medium and to establish the optimal exposure factors
15. Tangential, lateral, and axial (intraoral method) projections
16. c
17. c
18. c
19. b
20. True
21. True
22. False (Only one parotid gland can be demonstrated with each tangential projection.)
23. a. Tangential projection
    b. Parotid
    c. The patient can fill his or her mouth with air and then puff the cheeks out as much as possible.
24. a. Lateral projection
    b. Parotid
    c. Parotid
25. a. Lateral projection
    b. Submandibular
    c. Submandibular

Self-Test: Mouth and Salivary Glands

1. a	5. b	9. c	13. a
2. a	6. d	10. d	14. c
3. b	7. b	11. a	15. b
4. a	8. a	12. a	

CHAPTER 15 **Anterior Part of the Neck**

Review

1. A. Nasal septum
   B. Nasopharynx
   C. Uvula
   D. Epiglottis
   E. Vocal folds
   F. Larynx
   G. Laryngeal pharynx
   H. Soft palate
   I. Piriform recess
   J. Rima glottidis
2. A. Soft palate
   B. Nasopharynx
   C. Uvula
   D. Oropharynx
   E. Epiglottis
   F. Vocal folds
   G. Larynx
   H. Hard palate
   I. Hyoid bone
   J. Laryngeal pharynx
   K. Trachea
   L. Thyroid cartilage
   M. Esophagus

3. A. Superior thyroid artery
   B. Superior parathyroid gland
   C. Thyroid gland
   D. Inferior parathyroid gland
   E. Esophagus
   F. Thyroid cartilage
   G. Isthmus of the thyroid
   H. Trachea
4. A. Hyoid bone
   B. Thyroid cartilage
   C. Trachea
5. A. Base of the tongue
   B. Epiglottis
   C. Vestibular fold (false vocal cord)
   D. Rima glottidis (open)
   E. Rima glottidis (closed)
   F. Vocal fold (true vocal cord)
6. Posterior; anterior
7. Trachea
8. Esophagus
9. Thyroid; parathyroid
10. Pharynx
11. Nasopharynx
12. Oropharynx
13. Larynx
14. Glottis
15. AP projection; lateral projection
16. Breathing, phonation, stress maneuvers, and swallowing
17. a. Supine
    b. Upright
18. Laryngeal prominence
19. a. Level of the external acoustic meatuses
    b. Level of the mandibular angles
    c. Level of the laryngeal prominence
20. A. Air-filled pharynx
    B. Hyoid bone
    C. Laryngeal structures
    D. Trachea

Self-Test: Anterior Part of the Neck

1. c	6. d
2. a	7. b
3. d	8. b
4. b	9. b
5. c	10. b

CHAPTER 16 **Digestive System: Abdomen, Liver, Spleen, and Biliary Tract**

SECTION 1 **Anatomy of the Abdomen, Liver, Spleen, and Biliary Tract**

Exercise 1

1. A. Right lobe of the liver
   B. Liver
   C. Gallbladder
   D. Ascending colon
   E. Ileum
   F. Cecum
   G. Veriform appendix
   H. Left lobe of the liver
   I. Pancreas
   J. Esophagus
   K. Stomach
   L. Spleen
   M. Left colic flexure
   N. Descending colon
   O. Transverse colon
   P. Small intestine
   Q. Sigmoid colon
   R. Urinary bladder
2. A. Tongue
   B. Sublingual gland
   C. Submandibular gland
   D. Gallbladder
   E. Biliary ducts
   F. Visceral surface of the liver
   G. Veriform appendix
   H. Parotid gland
   I. Pharynx
   J. Esophagus
   K. Stomach
   L. Spleen
   M. Pancreas
   N. Large intestine
   O. Small intestine
3. A. Hepatopancreatic ampulla
   B. Cystic duct
   C. Right lobe of the liver
   D. Gallbladder
   E. Liver
   F. Falciform ligament
   G. Quadrate lobe of the liver
   H. Left lobe of the liver
   I. Left hepatic duct
   J. Caudate lobe of the liver
   K. Common hepatic duct
   L. Common bile duct
   M. Pancreatic duct
   N. Pancreas
   O. Duodenum
4. A. Cut surface of the liver
   B. Gallbladder
   C. Cystic duct
   D. Right kidney
   E. Common hepatic duct
   F. Common bile duct
   G. Spleen
   H. Left kidney
   I. Pancreas
   J. Duodenum
5. A. Liver
   B. Inferior vena cava
   C. Right kidney
   D. Stomach
   E. Spleen
   F. Left kidney
   G. Aorta

Exercise 2

1. Peritoneum
2. Parietal; visceral
3. Parietal
4. Visceral
5. Liver
6. Liver
7. Bile
8. Common hepatic duct
9. Gallbladder
10. Liver
11. Common bile duct
12. Pancreatic duct
13. Cholecystokinin
14. Hepatopancreatic ampulla
15. Pancreas
16. True
17. False (The gallbladder is located on the inferior surface of the right lobe of the liver, within the abdominal cavity.)
18. True
19. True
20. True

SECTION 2 **Positioning of the Abdomen and Gallbladder**

Exercise 1: Positioning for the Abdomen

1. KUB
2. Iliac crests
3. 2 inches (5 cm) above the iliac crests (high enough to include the diaphragm) and to the level of the iliac crests (to include the bladder)
4. Gonadal shielding is desirable if the gonads lie within close proximity (2 inches [5 cm]) to the primary x-ray field; gonadal shielding should be used if the clinical objectives of the examination will not be compromised; and gonadal shielding should be used if the patient has a reasonable reproductive potential.
5. Psoas
6. Expiration
7. To allow the patient to come to rest and to allow the involuntary movement of the viscera to subside
8. Midsagittal
9. Diaphragm (to demonstrate any free air within the abdominal cavity that may rise and become trapped under the diaphragm)
10. A right or left marker and an appropriate marker indicating the patient is upright
11. A reduction in the radiation exposure to the gonads
12. Supine KUB, AP upright abdomen, and PA chest
13. To demonstrate abdominal free air that may accumulate under the diaphragm
14. Left lateral decubitus
15. b, d, e
16. Demonstration of air-fluid levels
17. To enable rising free air to be seen through the homogeneous background density of the liver instead of becoming superimposed with air in the stomach

18. The patient should be recumbent in a lateral position with the left side down (left lateral recumbent), both arms raised above the diaphragm, and the knees slightly flexed.
19. To allow any air to rise to its highest level within the abdomen
20. A vertically placed cassette should be centered against the patient's posterior side of the abdomen at the level of the iliac crests.
21. Suspend respiration after expiration.
22. Perpendicular (horizontally) to the midpoint of the cassette, entering at the level of the iliac crests
23. The "up" side
24. The dependent "down" side
25. Diaphragm
26. Markers indicating the side of the patient and which side is up
27. True
28. False (Make the exposure after the patient suspends respiration after expiration.)
29. False (The midcoronal plane should be perpendicular and centered to the cassette.)
30. The iliac crests (or high enough to ensure demonstration of the diaphragm)
31. Across the pelvis
32. To a point on the midcoronal plane at the level of the iliac crests
33. Pelvis and lumbar vertebrae
34. Dorsal decubitus
35. Midcoronal plane
36. 2 inches (5 cm)
37. To relieve strain on the patient's back by reducing the lordotic curvature
38. False (Make the exposure after the suspension of expiration.)
39. True
40. b, c, d

Exercise 2: Contrast Studies for the Gallbladder

1. Cholecystography
2. Oral
3. OCG; GB
4. Portal
5. a. The presence of stones or calculi in the gallbladder
   b. Calculi in the common bile duct
   c. An acute or chronic inflammation of the gallbladder
   d. A narrowing or occlusion of the common bile duct
6. Gallstones
7. Preliminary preparation of the intestinal tract; preliminary diet; exact time to swallow the oral tablets; avoidance of laxatives for 24 hours before swallowing the tablets; avoidance of all foods, both solids and liquids (except water), after swallowing the tablets; and the time to report for the examination
8. Vomiting or diarrhea may cause most of the contrast medium to be expelled from the patient, rendering a poorly and partially opacified gallbladder.
9. Prolonged fasting can cause the formation of gas, which could make it difficult to clearly visualize the gallbladder.
10. Preparation for an OCG examination can be shortened if the intestinal tract is found to be sufficiently clean, and radiopaque gallstones may be demonstrated before they can be obscured by the contrast medium.
11. To allow irritation of the intestinal tract mucosal lining to subside (this requires 24 hours) and to prevent the egestion of the contrast medium with the fecal material
12. Only small drinks of water
13. Ultrasonography

14. True
15. True
16. True
17. False (The right side of the abdomen should be centered to the midline of the table.)
18. Small
19. ½ second
20. Instruct the patient to spread the breasts superiorly and laterally to clear the gallbladder region.
21. To rotate the vertebrae slightly to the left
22. Elevate the ankles.
23. After the suspension of expiration
24. 2 seconds (to permit any peristaltic action to subside and to give the patient time to relax)
25. a. Fig. 16-11
    b. Fig. 16-12
26. Make the exposure after the patient suspends respiration after inspiration.
27. a. Sthenic
    b. Hypersthenic
    c. Asthenic
28. Lower
29. 2 to 4 inches (5 to 10 cm)
30. Within the fundic portion
31. a. *U*
    b. *U*
    c. *P*
    d. *U*
    e. *U*
    f. *P*
    g. *U*
    h. *P*
32. Vertebral column (Vertebrae or thoracic vertebrae are also acceptable.)
33. 15 to 40 degrees
34. The location of the gallbladder with reference to the vertebral column; the angulation of the long axis of the gallbladder; and whether the right colic flexure is clear or obscures the gallbladder
35. Thin
36. The LAO position places the gallbladder closer to the cassette.
37. To compress the viscera and thus help eliminate movement
38. Because the gallbladder is normally on the right side of the abdomen, a right lateral position places the gallbladder closer to the cassette than does a left lateral. (A left lateral position should be the position of choice if the patient's gallbladder is on the left side of the abdomen.)
39. Renal (kidney)
40. Expiration
41. Thin
42. Short-scale
43. Right
44. Below
45. Short
46. Decubitus
47. c
48. c
49. True
50. False (The mobility of the gallbladder often causes the organ to partially superimpose the vertebrae when the patient is placed in the left lateral position, thus making it difficult to clearly completely image the gallbladder without bony superimposition.)

Exercise 3: Identifying Gallbladder Radiographs

1. LAO
2. Right lateral decubitus
3. PA (prone)
4. PA (upright)

Self-Test: Abdomen, Liver, Spleen, and Biliary Tract

1. a	14. a	27. b	39. a
2. d	15. d	28. a	40. a
3. d	16. b	29. a	41. c
4. b	17. a	30. d	42. a
5. d	18. a	31. d	43. b
6. c	19. d	32. d	44. a
7. b	20. c	33. b	45. b
8. d	21. a	34. b	46. a
9. a	22. b	35. a	47. d
10. d	23. c	36. b	48. d
11. d	24. a	37. c	49. d
12. b	25. a	38. b	50. d
13. a	26. b		

CHAPTER 17 **Digestive System: Alimentary Canal**

SECTION 1 **Anatomy of the Alimentary Canal**

Exercise 1

1. A. Tongue
   B. Sublingual gland
   C. Submandibular gland
   D. Gallbladder
   E. Biliary ducts
   F. Veriform appendix
   G. Rectum
   H. Parotid gland
   I. Pharynx
   J. Esophagus
   K. Stomach
   L. Spleen
   M. Pancreas
   N. Large intestine
   O. Small intestine
2. A. Cardiac antrum
   B. Cardia
   C. Lesser curvature
   D. Angular notch
   E. Pyloric sphincter
   F. Duodenum
   G. Pyloric canal
   H. Pyloric antrum
   I. Greater curvature
   J. Cardiac notch
   K. Fundus
   L. Body
3. A. Cardiac sphincter
   B. Pyloric sphincter
   C. Duodenum
   D. Pyloric canal
   E. Rugae

4. A. Greater duodenal papilla (orifice of biliary and pancreatic ducts)
   B. Hepatopancreatic ampulla
   C. Gallbladder
   D. Cystic duct
   E. Common hepatic duct
   F. Common bile duct
   G. Pylorus
   H. Stomach
   I. Pancreatic duct
   J. Pancreas
   K. Duodenum
5. A. Ileum
   B. Veriform appendix
   C. Cecum
   D. Ascending colon
   E. Right colic flexure
   F. Transverse colon
   G. Left colic flexure
   H. Descending colon
   I. Sigmoid colon
   J. Rectum
6. A. Sacrum
   B. Anal canal
   C. Rectum
   D. Rectal ampulla

Exercise 2

Exercise 3

1. b	6. c	11. b	16. a
2. a	7. a	12. c	17. b
3. a	8. a	13. c	18. a
4. b	9. c	14. c	19. c
5. c	10. b	15. a	20. c

Exercise 4

1. Esophagus
2. Cardiac antrum
3. Cardiac orifice
4. Stomach
5. Rugae
6. Right (medial)
7. Pylorus
8. Greater curvature
9. a. Hypersthenic
   b. Sthenic
   c. Hyposthenic
   d. Asthenic
10. Cardia, fundus, body, and pylorus
11. Cardia
12. Fundus
13. Pyloric
14. Pyloric orifice
15. Duodenum; jejunum; ileum
16. Duodenum
17. Duodenal bulb
18. Ileocecal valve
19. Duodenum
20. Jejunum
21. Ileum
22. Duodenum; ileum
23. Small
24. Ileocecal valve
25. Cecum
26. Cecum
27. Right colic
28. Ascending
29. Transverse
30. Left colic
31. Descending
32. Descending colon; rectum
33. Rectum
34. Anal canal
35. Anus

SECTION 2 Positioning of the Alimentary Canal

Exercise 1: Positioning for the Esophagus

1. AP (or PA) projection, oblique (RAO or LPO) projection, and lateral projection
2. A high-density barium product and carbon dioxide crystals
3. The LAO projection may superimpose vertebral shadows with the distal esophagus
4. T5 to T6 (top of cassette should be centered to the mouth)
5. RAO and LPO
6. It allows more complete contrast filling of the esophagus
7. the esophagus should be adequately demonstrated through the superimposed thoracic vertebrae
8. To the left of the vertebral column, between the thoracic vertebrae and the heart
9. Partially obscured by thoracic vertebrae
10. Posterior ribs should be superimposed

11. 35 degrees; 40 degrees
12. Cardiac orifice
13. True
14. True
15. False (a 30% to 50% weight per volume suspension is acceptable. The most important criterion for the barium is that the flow must be sufficient to coat esophageal walls.)

Exercise 2: The Gastrointestinal Series

1. GI and UGI
2. To reduce the production of intestinal gas and fecal material
3. The coating ability of the barium could be diminished because the secretion of gastric juices may be stimulated.
4. A barium sulfate product of 30% to 50% weight per volume concentration
5. Single-contrast examination and double-contrast examination
6. 30% to 50%
7. High-density barium sulfate suspension and gas-producing substance
8. Small lesions are readily demonstrated and the mucosal lining of the stomach can be more clearly visualized.
9. False (The examination should begin with the patient upright.)
10. True
11. False (Most radiographs are obtained with the patient in the recumbent position to provide better coating of the mucosal surface.)
12. To coat the mucosal lining of the stomach
13. To relax the gastric tract, enabling gastric structures to expand and thus be better demonstrated
14. The patient should be instructed not to belch.
15. A biphasic GI examination is a UGI examination in which the patient is first examined with a double-contrast procedure, after which a low weight per volume barium sulfate suspension is administered and the patient is examined with a single-contrast procedure
16. Double-contrast
17. With intubation and without intubation
18. True
19. True
20. True
21. False (The patient should be in the recumbent position.)
22. True
23. True
24. False (A compression band should not be used to immobilize the patient, because its use can cause filling defects and interfere with the filling and emptying of the duodenal bulb.)
25. The patient's weight should be supported by cushions placed under the thorax and pelvis.
26. To midway between the vertebral column and the lateral border of the abdomen at the level of L1-L2
27. To the midsagittal plane at the level of L1-L2
28. Center the cassette 3 to 6 inches (7.5 to 15 cm) lower.
29. Asthenic
30. L1-L2
31. Expiration
32. Instruct the patient to turn toward the left, elevating the left side away from the x-ray table, and to support the raised left side with the left forearm and flexed left knee.
33. On the left side of the abdomen, midway between the vertebral column and the lateral border of the abdomen at the level of L1-L2
34. c
35. c

36. True
37. False (The patient should suspend respiration after expiration.)
38. Supine
39. Right
40. 45 degrees
41. On the left side of the abdomen, midway between the vertebral column and the lateral border of the abdomen, at the level of L1-L2
42. True
43. False (An air-contrast image, not a barium-filled image, of the pyloric canal and duodenal bulb is produced with the LPO position.)
44. A. Distal esophagus
   B. Fundus
   C. Body
   D. Pylorus
   E. Duodenum
45. b
46. b
47. c
48. b
49. a. Gas-filled
   b. Barium-filled
   c. Barium-filled
50. A. Fundus
   B. Body
   C. Duodenum
   D. Duodenal bulb
   E. Pyloric portion
51. a. Midway between the vertebral column and the left lateral border of the abdomen at the level of L1/L2
   b. To the midsagittal plane at the level of L1/L2
52. b
53. d
54. a. Gas-filled (double-contrast)
   b. Barium-filled
   c. Gas-filled (double-contrast)
   d. Gas-filled (double-contrast)
55. A. Fundus
   B. Body
   C. Pyloric portion
   D. Duodenal loop

Exercise 3: Small Intestine Examination

1. Orally, reflux filling, and intubation (direct injection)
2. a
3. c
4. b
5. b
6. c
7. a, b, f, g
8. c
9. a
10. b
11. b
12. To indicate the interval between the exposure of the radiograph and the ingestion of the barium
13. By accelerating peristalsis
14. c
15. b
16. b
17. c

18. a
19. a
20. a, b, d, e, f, h, i

Exercise 4: Large Intestine Examination

1. c
2. Barium sulfate
3. To obtain better coating of the lumen
4. Air and carbon dioxide
5. When the patient cannot tolerate retrograde filling of the colon
6. Although it may vary, typical preparation includes a restrictive diet, laxatives, and a cleansing enema
7. The entire colon should be as clean as possible; no fecal material should be present.
8. Approximately 85-90° F
9. Barium that is too warm may be unpleasant and debilitating to the patient, may injure internal tissues, and may produce irritation that makes it difficult for the patient to retain the barium for as long as required.
10. Approximately 41° F
11. Cold barium causes less irritation to the colon, relaxes the colon, and stimulates tonal contraction of the anal sphincter to increase patient comfort, facilitate better toleration of the examination, and improve retention of the barium.
12. Maintain tight contraction of the anal sphincter around the enema tip, relax the abdominal muscles, and concentrate on deep oral breathing.
13. c
14. b
15. Postevacuation
16. a
17. c
18. a
19. A. Left colic flexure
    B. Right colic flexure
    C. Transverse colon
    D. Descending colon
    E. Ascending colon
    F. Cecum
    G. Sigmoid
    H. Rectum
20. c
21. b
22. c
23. b
24. False (Superior colic structures [transverse colon and both flexures] need not be demonstrated.)
25. A. Left colic flexure
    B. Transverse colon
    C. Sigmoid
    D. Rectum
26. False (The central ray should be directed perpendicular to the center of the cassette.)
27. True
28. True
29. True
30. A. Left colic flexure
    B. Right colic flexure
    C. Descending colon
    D. Ascending colon
    E. Sigmoid

31. c
32. b
33. A. Left colic flexure
    B. Right colic flexure
    C. Transverse colon
    D. Descending colon
    E. Ascending colon
    F. Veriform appendix
    G. Sigmoid
34. To the level of the anterior superior iliac spines
35. Hips and femurs should be superimposed.
36. a
37. c
38. A. Sigmoid
    B. Sacrum
    C. Rectum
    D. Pubic symphysis
39. Midsagittal
40. Iliac crests
41. True
42. True
43. A. Left colic (spenic) flexure
    B. Transverse colon
    C. Right colic flexure
    D. Descending colon
    E. Ascending colon
    F. Sigmoid
44. b
45. d
46. 2 inches (5 cm) below the level of the anterior superior iliac spines
47. The inferior margin of the pubic symphysis
48. A. Descending colon
    B. Sigmoid
    C. Rectum
49. PA oblique; RAO
50. 35 degrees; 45 degrees
51. Right
52. Right colic
53. A. Left colic flexure
    B. Right colic flexure
    C. Descending colon
    D. Ascending colon
    E. Sigmoid
    F. Rectum
54. LAO
55. Left colic
56. 35 to 45 degrees
57. A. Left colic flexure
    B. Transverse colon
    C. Right colic flexure
    D. Descending colon
    E. Ascending colon
    F. Sigmoid
58. b
59. Support the patient on a radiolucent pad.
60. Area from the flexures to the rectum
61. a. Right lateral decubitus
    b. Left lateral decubitus

62. a. Fig. 17-37
    b. Fig. 17-36
    c. Fig. 17-36
    d. Fig. 17-37
    e. Fig. 17-37
    f. Fig. 17-36
63. It is lower—generally 2 to 3 inches (5 to 7.5 cm)—because of the gravitational effect.
64. a. Upright
    b. Liquid barium can be seen settling to the lower levels of the colon.
65. 1. g
    2. c
    3. e
    4. d
    5. a
    6. b
    7. f
    8. h

Self-Test: Anatomy and Positioning of the Alimentary Canal

1. d	14. c	27. d	39. b
2. a	15. a	28. d	40. c
3. c	16. c	29. d	41. a
4. d	17. b	30. d	42. c
5. d	18. d	31. a	43. c
6. b	19. b	32. b	44. b
7. d	20. b	33. c	45. c
8. d	21. a	34. c	46. b
9. a	22. c	35. b	47. b
10. b	23. c	36. b	48. b
11. b	24. d	37. c	49. b
12. d	25. b	38. d	50. b
13. c	26. b		

CHAPTER 18 Urinary System
SECTION 1 Anatomy of the Urinary System

Exercise 1

1. A. Right kidney
   B. Inferior vena cava
   C. Aorta
   D. Left kidney
   E. Left ureter
   F. Urinary bladder
2. A. Right kidney
   B. Right ureter
   C. Urinary bladder
   D. Rectum
   E. Prostate
   F. Anal canal

3. A. Hilum
   B. Renal papilla
   C. Renal pelvis
   D. Renal cortex
   E. Renal sinus
   F. Renal medulla
   G. Renal pyramid
   H. Minor calyx
   I. Major calyx
4. A. Cortex
   B. Medulla
   C. Afferent arteriole
   D. Efferent arteriole
   E. Glomerulus
   F. Distal convoluted tubule
   G. Glomerular capsule
   H. Proximal convoluted tubule
   I. Descending limb of Henle's loop
   J. Ascending limb of Henle's loop
   K. Collecting duct
5. A. Ovary
   B. Uterine tube
   C. Uterus
   D. Bladder
   E. Pubic symphysis
   F. Urethra
   G. Vagina
   H. Rectum
6. A. Bladder
   B. Pubic symphysis
   C. Urethra
   D. Sacrum
   E. Rectum
   F. Prostate

Exercise 2

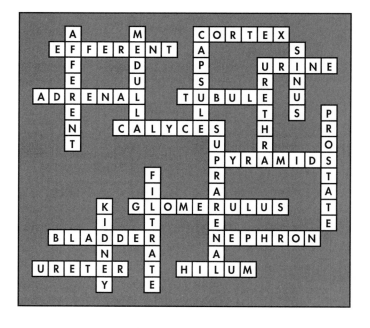

Exercise 3

1. Urinary
2. Kidney
3. Suprarenal
4. Hilum
5. Medial
6. T12
7. Nephron
8. Cortex
9. Glomerular
10. Glomerulus
11. Renal
12. Afferent; efferent
13. Glomerular filtrate
14. Calyces
15. Calyces
16. Pelvis
17. Ureters
18. Urinary bladder
19. Urethra
20. Prostate

Exercise 4: Venipuncture and IV Contrast Media Administration

1. b
2. a
3. b
4. c
5. c
6. a
7. Inject into the bottle an amount of air equal to the amount of fluid to be withdrawn.
8. A pulse indicates the vessel is an artery.
9. b, d, g, h
10. Using tincture of iodine 1%-2% or isopropyl 70%, wipe the skin with a circular motion covering an area that is approximately 2 inches in diameter without lifting the swab from the skin until the process is completed.
11. 6 to 8 inches
12. Bevel-up
13. 45 degrees
14. The vein has been successfully penetrated by the needle.
15. Remove the needle and apply direct pressure to the puncture site.
16. c
17. c
18. b
19. a, b, c, d
20. a, b, c, e, f

SECTION 2 Positioning of the Urinary System

Exercise 1: Excretory Urography

1. Urography
2. d
3. a, b, c, e
4. a, c, e, f, i, k
5. a
6. a, c, e, g

7. To distend the stomach with gas, thus providing a negative background density that better demonstrates renal structures
8. Inappropriate abdominal pressure might retard the excretion of fluid from the kidneys and might cause distortion of ureteral structures.
9. To retard the flow of opacified urine into the bladder, allowing renal structures to be better filled and demonstrated
10. The anterior surface of the lower abdomen, about 2 inches (5 cm) above the pubic symphysis
11. Rapid releasing of the ureteral compression device might rupture some of the viscera within the pelvis.
12. Increased doses of contrast agents and the use of contrast media of higher concentrations produce better demonstration of ureters.
13. To demonstrate the mobility of the kidneys
14. Patient data, side marker, time-interval, and position indicator
15. Elastic waistbands in the underwear can produce unwanted densities in the image because of soft tissue skin folds.
16. c
17. b, c, d, e, h
18. d
19. a
20. b
21. c
22. b
23. True
24. True
25. False (Postinjection radiographs are most often obtained with the patient supine.)
26. d
27. d
28. d
29. a
30. c
31. d
32. A. Renal calyces
    B. Renal pelvis
    C. Abdominal ureter
    D. Pelvic ureter
    E. Urinary bladder
33. b
34. Left
35. c
36. c
37. b
38. a
39. Midcornal
40. Arms extended in front of the patient, elbows flexed, and hands placed under the head
41. Pelvis and lumbar vertebrae
42. Expiration
43. Short
44. Supine
45. Midcoronal
46. a
47. b
48. True
49. False (The exposure should be made at the end of expiration.)
50. True

Exercise 2: Retrograde Urography

1. False (Contrast agents are injected into a selected renal pelvis by means of catheters that pass through the urethra, the bladder, and the ureter to the selected kidney.)
2. False (Special cystoscopic-radiographic tables are used for retrograde studies.)
3. c
4. c
5. a
6. The urologist intravenously injects a color dye, and the function of each kidney is determined by the time required for the dye substance to appear in the urine as it passes through the respective catheter.
7. A preliminary radiograph showing catheter insertion, a pyelogram, and a ureterogram
8. By retarding the excretion of the contrast medium from the kidney, the filling of the renal pelvis is enhanced.
9. b
10. a

Exercise 3: Retrograde Cystography

1. By means of a catheter passed through the urethra into the bladder
2. d
3. b
4. c
5. c
6. b
7. b
8. b
9. a
10. b
11. c
12. b
13. c
14. c
15. a, b
16. Above
17. Lateral recumbent
18. Pubic symphysis
19. b
20. c

Exercise 4: Male Cystourethrography

1. The radiographic examination of the urinary bladder and urethra after the introduction of a contrast medium by means of a catheter inserted into the bladder
2. A catheter is inserted through the urethral canal into the bladder.
3. d
4. c
5. d
6. True
7. True
8. True
9. False (Only the bladder and urethra need to be demonstrated in their entirety.)
10. True

Exercise 5: Identifying Urinary System Radiographs

1. d
2. a
3. b
4. b
5. a
6. b
7. a
8. a
9. b
10. d

Self-Test: Anatomy and Positioning of the Urinary System

1. a	8. b	14. b	20. a
2. b	9. c	15. d	21. c
3. c	10. d	16. b	22. a
4. b	11. a	17. b	23. c
5. d	12. b	18. c	24. d
6. c	13. a	19. d	25. d
7. c			

CHAPTER 19 Reproductive System
SECTION 1 Anatomy of the Reproductive System

Exercise 1

1. A. Fundus
   B. Round ligament
   C. Ovarian ligament
   D. Uterine tube
   E. Ovary
2. A. Uterine tube (cut)
   B. Cervix
   C. Uterine ostium
   D. Rectum
   E. Ovary
   F. Uterine tube
   G. Uterus
   H. Round ligament (cut)
   I. Urinary bladder
   J. Pubic symphysis
   K. Urethral orifice
   L. Vaginal orifice
3. Ovaries
4. Ova
5. Uterine (or fallopian)
6. Two
7. Uterus
8. Fundus, body, isthmus, and cervix
9. Cervix
10. 1. e
    2. a
    3. b
    4. d
    5. c

Exercise 2

1. A. Testicular artery
   B. Ductus deferens
   C. Epididymis
   D. Head of the epididymis
   E. Testis
2. A. Sacrum
   B. Rectum
   C. Prostate
   D. Testes
   E. Bladder
   F. Pubis
   G. Urethra
3. A. Ureter
   B. Ductus deferens
   C. Bladder
   D. Seminal vesicle
   E. Ampulla
   F. Prostate
   G. Epididymis
   H. Testis
4. Testes (or testicles)
5. Spermatozoa
6. Epididymis
7. Ductus deferens
8. Ejaculatory
9. Prostate
10. Urethra

SECTION 2 **Radiography of the Reproductive System**

Exercise 1: Radiography of the Female Reproductive System

1. 1. a
   2. a
   3. b
   4. a
   5. b
   6. b
2. 1. b
   2. b
   3. d
   4. e
   5. c, e, f
   6. c, f
   7. f
   8. a, b, d, e
   9. a, b
   10. c
   11. f
   12. e
   13. c, e, f
   14. f
   15. c

3. i. d
   ii. c
   iii. b
   iv. b
   v. a

Exercise 2: Radiography of the Male Reproductive System

1. Water-soluble, iodinated
2. To improve radiographic contrast of examined structures
3. Prostate
4. Prone (because it places the prostate closer to the cassette and the sacrococcygeal vertebrae farther from the cassette)
5. 20 to 25 degrees cephalad

Self-Test: Reproductive System

1. a	6. c	11. d
2. c	7. c	12. b
3. b	8. a	13. b
4. a	9. d	14. c
5. b	10. d	15. b

CHAPTER 20 **Skull**

SECTION 1 **Osteology of the Skull**

Exercise 1

1. A. Parietal bone
   B. Glabella
   C. Greater wing of the sphenoid
   D. Nasal bone
   E. Temporal bone
   F. Zygomatic bone
   G. Perpendicular plate of the ethmoid
   H. Vomer
   I. Maxilla
   J. Frontal bone
   K. Sphenoid bone
   L. Lacrimal bone
   M. Ethmoid bone
   N. Middle nasal concha
   O. Infraorbital foramen
   P. Inferior nasal concha
   Q. Anterior nasal spine
   R. Mandible

2. A. Frontal bone
   B. Sphenoid bone
   C. Glabella
   D. Nasal bone
   E. Lacrimal bone
   F. Ethmoid bone
   G. Anterior nasal spine (acanthion)
   H. Zygomatic bone (zygoma)
   I. Zygomatic arch
   J. Maxilla
   K. Mental foramen
   L. Mandible
   M. Bregma
   N. Coronal suture
   O. Parietal bone
   P. Squamosal suture
   Q. Lambda
   R. Lambdoidal suture
   S. Occipital bone
   T. External occipital protuberance (inion)
   U. Mastoid process
   V. Temporal bone
   W. External acoustic meatus
   X. Styloid process

3. A. Orbital plate
   B. Lesser wing
   C. Greater wing
   D. Optic groove
   E. Foramen ovale
   F. Foramen spinosum
   G. Temporal bone
   H. Petrous portion
   I. Clivus
   J. Occipital bone
   K. Crista galli
   L. Cribriform plate
   M. Optic canal and foramen
   N. Tuberculum sellae
   O. Anterior clinoid process
   P. Sella turcica
   Q. Posterior clinoid process
   R. Foramen lacerum
   S. Dorsum sellae
   T. Jugular foramen
   U. Hypoglossal canal
   V. Foramen magnum

4. A. Frontal bone
   B. Frontal sinus
   C. Crista galli
   D. Nasal bone
   E. Ethmoid bone
   F. Vomer
   G. Maxilla
   H. Parietal bone
   I. Sphenoidal sinus
   J. Petrous portion
   K. Internal acoustic meatus
   L. Occipital bone
   M. Squamous portion of the temporal bone
   N. Clivus
   O. Pterygoid hamulus
   P. Palatine bone

5. A. Frontal squama
   B. Supraorbital foramen
   C. Supraorbital margin
   D. Glabella
   E. Nasal spine
   F. Superciliary arch
   G. Frontal eminence

6. A. Superior nasal conchar
   B. Middle nasal concha
   C. Perpendicular plate
   D. Crista galli
   E. Ethmoidal sinus
   F. Air cells in the labyrinth
   G. Cribriform plate

7. A. Parietal
   B. Frontal
   C. Frontal
   D. Sphenoid
   E. Occipital
   F. Occipital
   G. Mastoid
   H. Temporal

8. A. Anterior clinoid processes
   B. Posterior clinoid processes
   C. Dorsum sellae
   D. Lateral pterygoid lamina
   E. Pterygoid hamulus
   F. Optic canal and foramen
   G. Lesser wing
   H. Superior orbital fissure
   I. Greater wing

9. A. Squama
   B. Foramen magnum
   C. Basilar portion
   D. Occipital condyle
   E. External occipital protuberance (inion)

10. A. Squamous portion
    B. Mastoid portion
    C. External acoustic meatus
    D. Tympanic portion
    E. Styloid process
    F. Mandibular fossa
    G. Articular tubercle
    H. Zygomatic process
    I. Petrous portion

11. A. External acoustic meatus
    B. Cartilage
    C. Tympanic membrane
    D. Auditory ossicles
    E. Semicircular canals
    F. Stapes (in oval window)
    G. Internal acoustic meatus
    H. Cochlear nerve
    I. Cochlea
    J. Round window
    K. Auditory (Eustachian) tube
    L. Nasopharynx
    M. External acoustic meatus
    N. Auditory tube

12. A. Neck
    B. Condyle
    C. Alveolar process
    D. Mental foramen
    E. Symphysis
    F. Coronoid process
    G. Ramus
    H. Body
    I. Mental protuberance
    J. Angle
    K. Gonion
13. A. Body
    B. Greater cornu
    C. Lesser cornu

Exercise 2

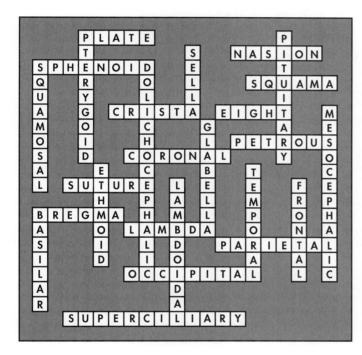

Exercise 3

1. a
2. a
3. c
4. d
5. d
6. f
7. b
8. d
9. f
10. b
11. e
12. f
13. e
14. d
15. e
16. a
17. b
18. d
19. d
20. d

Exercise 4

1. m
2. q
3. i
4. c
5. e
6. n
7. r
8. l
9. k
10. p
11. g
12. j
13. f
14. b
15. s

Exercise 5

1. Cranial; facial
2. Frontal (1); ethmoid (1); parietal (2); sphenoid (1); temporal (2); and occipital (1)
3. Nasal (2); lacrimal (2); maxillae (2); zygomatic (2); palatine (2); inferior nasal conchae (2); vomer (1); and mandible (1)
4. Flat
5. Diploe
6. Bregma; lambda
7. Bregma
8. Lambda
9. Mesocephalic (47 degrees); brachycephalic (54 degrees); and dolichocephalic (40 degrees)
10. Frontal
11. Ethmoid
12. Parietal
13. Eminence
14. Sagittal
15. Coronal
16. Occipital
17. Lambdoidal
18. Sphenoid
19. Occipital
20. Basilar
21. Foramen magnum
22. Sphenoid
23. C1 vertebra (atlas)
24. Sphenoid
25. Temporal
26. Tympanic
27. Mastoid
28. Petrous portion (pars petrosa, petrous pyramid)
29. Temporal
30. Auricle
31. Malleus (hammer); incus (anvil); stapes (stirrup)
32. Temporal
33. Temporal
34. Nasal
35. Lacrimal
36. Maxilla
37. Maxillary sinus

38. Alveolar process
39. Maxillae
40. Acanthion
41. Zygomatic
42. Zygomatic
43. Palatine
44. Inferior nasal conchae
45. Vomer
46. Mandible
47. Ramus
48. Hyoid
49. Condyle; coronoid
50. Condyle

SECTION 2 Radiography of the Skull

Exercise 1: Skull Topography

1. A. Angle of the mandible (gonion)
   B. Infraorbitomeatal margin
   C. Outer canthus
   D. Midsagittal plane
   E. Glabella
   F. Interpupillary line
   G. Inner canthus
   H. Nasion
   I. Acanthion
   J. Mental point
2. A. External acoustic meatus
   B. Angle of the mandible (gonion)
   C. Glabellomeatal line
   D. Orbitomeatal line
   E. Infraorbitomeatal line
   F. Acanthiomeatal line
   G. Glabelloalveolar line
   H. Glabella
   I. Nasion
   J. Acanthion
   K. Mental point
3. 1. c
   2. f
   3. a
   4. e
   5. h
   6. d
   7. b
   8. i
   9. g
4. 1. e
   2. b
   3. h
   4. d
   5. i
   6. g
   7. f
5. a. 7
   b. 8

Exercise 2: Positioning for the Cranium

1. c
2. a. Parallel
   b. Perpendicular
3. c
4. d
5. 2 inches (5 cm) above the external acoustic meatus
6. Perpendicular to a point approximately 2 inches (5 cm) above the external acoustic meatus
7. a
8. False (The central ray should enter at a point 2 inches [5 cm] superior to the external acoustic meatus.)
9. True
10. b, c, d, e, f, g, h, j
11. a. A support should be placed under the thorax to raise the inferior aspect of the head and to place the midsagittal plane parallel with the cassette.
    b. A radiolucent sponge should be placed under the head to make the midsagittal plane parallel with the cassette.
12. A. Orbital roof
    B. Sella turcica
    C. Sphenoidal sinus
    D. Petrous portion of the temporal bone
    E. Temporomandibular joint
    F. External acoustic meatus
    G. Mandibular rami
13. a. Perpendicular
    b. Perpendicular
14. c
15. 1. a
    2. b
    3. d
    4. c
16. Nasion
17. Nasion
18. Stop breathing.
19. a, c, g, h, i
20. A. Dorsum sellae
    B. Superior orbital shadow (margin)
    C. Sphenoid plane
    D. Petrous ridge
    E. Ethmoidal sinus
    F. Inferior orbital shadow (margin)
    G. Crista galli
21. a. Perpendicular
    b. Perpendicular
22. Perpendicularly
23. Cephalically
24. a
25. c
26. a, c, g, h, j
27. a. 15 degrees cephalad (The petrous ridges lie in the lower one third of the orbits.)
    b. Perpendicularly (The petrous ridges fill the orbits.)
28. d
29. c
30. Orbitomeatal; infraorbitomeatal
31. a
32. c

33. Which positioning line (orbitomeatal or infraorbitomeatal) is perpendicular to the cassette
34. b, f, g, i
35. A. Parietal bone
    B. Occipital bone
    C. Foramen magnum
    D. Petrous ridge
    E. Posterior clinoid process
    F. Dorsum sellae
36. True
37. False (Hypersthenic patients must be either prone or upright.)
38. c
39. a
40. b
41. c
42. a, c, g, i
43. A. Occipital bone
    B. Foramen magnum
    C. Petrous ridge
    D. Posterior clinoid process
    E. Dorsum sellae
44. a. Perpendicular
    b. Parallel
45. Infraorbitomeatal
46. On the midsagittal plane of the throat between the angles of the mandible, passing through a point ¾ inch (2 cm) anterior to the level of the external acoustic meatus
47. a
48. b, e
49. a, d, f, h, i
50. A. Maxillary sinus
    B. Ethmoidal sinuses
    C. Mandible
    D. Sphenoidal sinus
    E. Foramen spinosum
    F. Mandibular condyle
    G. Dens (odontoid process)
    H. Petrosa
    I. Mastoid process

Exercise 3: Positioning for the Sella Turcica

1. a. Parallel
   b. Perpendicular
   c. Parallel
2. At a point ¾ inch (2 cm) anterior to and ¾ inch (2 cm) superior to the external acoustic meatus
3. Stop breathing.
4. a, b, c, d
5. A. Anterior clinoid process
   B. Posterior clinoid process
   C. Dorsum sellae
   D. Sella turcica
   E. Sphenoidal sinus

Exercise 4: Positioning for the Optic Canal and Foramen

1. b
2. b
3. a
4. True

5. True
6. False (The central ray should be directed perpendicularly through the affected orbit closer to the cassette.)
7. True
8. False (Incorrect angulation of the acanthiomeatal line causes longitudinal deviation from the preferred location of the optic canal and foramen. Any lateral deviation from the preferred location for the optic canal and foramen is caused by incorrect rotation of the head.)
9. b, e, f, g
10. A. Superior orbital margin
    B. Lateral orbital margin
    C. Optic canal and foramen
    D. Medial orbital margin
    E. Lesser wing of the sphenoid
    F. Ethmoidal sinus
    G. Inferior orbital margin
11. True
12. True
13. False (The orbitoparietal oblique projection is the AP oblique projection for the orbit. The PA oblique projection for the orbit is the parieto-orbital oblique projection.)
14. False (The orbitoparietal oblique projection results in more radiation exposure to the lens of the eye than the parieto-orbital oblique projection.)
15. True
16. Acanthiomeatal line
17. Midsagittal
18. a
19. b
20. c, e, f, g

Exercise 5: Evaluating Radiographs of the Skull

1. a. Fig. 20-38 (Certain structures of the skull are superimposed with their opposite side [orbital roofs, mandibular rami, mastoid regions, external acoustic meatuses, and temporomandibular joints], and no rotation is visible.)
   b. Fig. 20-37 (Cranial structures [orbital roofs, temporomandibular joints, and external acoustic meatuses] are longitudinally separated.)
   c. Fig. 20-36 (Cranial structures [orbital roofs, temporomandibular joints, and external acoustic meatuses] are laterally separated.)
   d. Fig. 20-37
2. a. Caudally 15 degrees
   b. In the lower one third of the orbits
   c. The distance from the lateral border of the skull to the lateral border of the orbit is not equal on both sides.
   d. The head is rotated, moving the occipital bone closer to the left shoulder. The midsagittal plane is not perpendicular to the cassette.
3. a. Perpendicular to the nasion
   b. The petrous ridges should fill the orbits.
   c. Yes
   d. The distance from the lateral border of the skull to the lateral border of the orbit is not equal on both sides.
   e. The head is rotated, moving the occipital bone closer to the right shoulder. The midsagittal plane is not perpendicular to the cassette.

4. a. Acceptable
   b. Unacceptable
   c. The head is rotated, moving the occipital bone closer to the left shoulder. The midsagittal plane is not perpendicular to the cassette.
   d. Perpendicularly
5. The mandibular symphysis does not superimpose the anterior frontal bone.
6. a. Fig. 20-45 (The optic foramen is demonstrated in the inferior and lateral quadrant of the orbit.)
   b. Fig. 20-44 (The position of the optic foramen is posterior to the lateral orbital margin.)
   c. Fig. 20-46 (The position of the optic foramen is too much toward the medial aspect of the orbit.)
7. a. The position of the optic foramen is deviated laterally from the preferred location.
   b. The angle formed by the midsagittal plane and the cassette was less than the required 53 degrees.
   c. Rotate the head, moving the occipital bone away from the cassette until the midsagittal plane forms an angle of 53 degrees with the cassette.

Self-Test: Osteology and Radiography of the Skull

1. a	19. b	37. a	54. a
2. d	20. c	38. d	55. d
3. a	21. d	39. c	56. d
4. b	22. b	40. b	57. c
5. c	23. a	41. d	58. d
6. d	24. b	42. d	59. c
7. d	25. a	43. b	60. d
8. d	26. c	44. c	61. a
9. b	27. d	45. b	62. b
10. a	28. c	46. c	63. d
11. c	29. b	47. a	64. d
12. d	30. d	48. a	65. c
13. a	31. b	49. c	66. c
14. c	32. d	50. c	67. b
15. a	33. b	51. a	68. c
16. b	34. c	52. c	69. c
17. a	35. c	53. d	70. b
18. c	36. c		

CHAPTER 21 Facial Bones
Radiography of the Facial Bones

Exercise 1: Positioning for Facial Bones and Nasal Bones

1. Lengthwise
2. Midsagittal
3. b
4. d
5. d
6. Perpendicularly
7. Halfway between the outer canthus and the EAM
8. a, b, d, g

9. A. Frontal sinus
   B. Nasal bone
   C. Sella turcica
   D. Maxillary sinus
   E. External acoustic meatus
   F. Maxilla
   G. Mandible
10. a. 37-degree angulation
    b. Perpendicular
11. b
12. a
13. a. Too far below maxillae (the maxillae will appear foreshortened)
    b. Immediately below the maxillae
    c. Superimpose maxillary sinuses
14. d, e
15. A. Orbit
    B. Zygomatic arch
    C. Maxillary sinus
    D. Maxilla
    E. Petrous ridge
    F. Mandibular angle
16. Supine
17. Parietoacanthial; Waters
18. b
19. c
20. a
21. a
22. c
23. d, e
24. A. Orbit
    B. Zygomatic bone
    C. Maxillary sinus
25. a. Perpendicular
    b. Parallel
26. Two
27. Nasion
28. Perpendicular to the bridge of the nose at a point ½ inch (1.2 cm) distal to the nasion
29. c, d
30. A. Frontonasal (nasofrontal)
    B. Nasal bone
    C. Anterior nasal spine of the maxilla

Exercise 2: Positioning for Zygomatic Arches

1. True
2. False (The zygomatic arches should be free from overlying structures.)
3. False (The posterior cranium need not be included in the image.)
4. False (The midsagittal plane should be perpendicular to the cassette.)
5. c
6. c
7. c
8. a
9. a, b, d
10. True
11. True
12. Infraorbitomeatal

13. Perpendicularly to the infraorbitomeatal line and centered to the zygomatic arch at a point approximately $1\frac{1}{2}$ inches (4 cm) posterior to the outer canthus
14. b
15. a. Perpendicular
    b. Perpendicular
16. a. 30 degrees caudad
    b. 37 degrees caudad
17. Nasion
18. True
19. False (Close beam restriction to zygomatic arches and adjacent structures may exclude the vertex.)
20. A. Occipital bone
    B. Mandible
    C. Zygomatic arch

Exercise 3: Positioning for the Mandible

1. b
2. a
3. Perpendicular
4. Stop breathing for the exposure.
5. b
6. b
7. True
8. False (The central portion of the mandible is superimposed with the cervical vertebrae.)
9. a, c
10. A. Condyle
    B. Mastoid process
    C. Fracture of the mandibular ramus
    D. Body
11. b
12. c
13. a
14. c
15. d
16. a
17. a, c, d
18. Fig. 21-18
19. Fig. 21-16
20. Fig. 21-18
21. Fig. 21-17
22. Fig. 21-16
23. Fig. 21- 17
24. Fig. 21-17
25. NA
26. Figs. 21-16, 21-17, and 21-18
27. NA
28. NA
29. Figs. 21-16, 21-17, and 21-18
30. Fig. 21-18
31. Fig. 21-16
32. True
33. False (The neck should be extended to place the mandibular body parallel with the transverse axis of the cassette.)
34. True

35. A. Coronoid process
    B. Mandibular condyle
    C. Ramus
    D. Body
    E. Mandibular angle (gonion)
    F. Hyoid bone

Exercise 4: Positioning for the Temporomandibular Joints (TMJs)

1. True
2. False (The head should be positioned the same way as for an AP projection, with the midsagittal plane perpendicular to the plane of the cassette.)
3. Occlusion of the incisors places the mandible in a position of protrusion in which the condyles are carried out of the mandibular fossae.
4. Any trauma to the mandible where the mandible is suspected to be fractured; because of the danger of fracture displacement
5. c
6. c
7. c
8. c
9. a, c
10. a, d
11. c
12. c
13. c
14. 15 degrees caudad
15. The TMJ closer to the cassette
16. In the mandibular fossa
17. False (To exit through the EAM closest to the cassette, the caudally directed central ray should enter about $1\frac{1}{2}$ inches [4 cm] superior to the upside EAM.)
18. True
19. False (Close beam restriction should surround the affected TMJ.)
20. A. Mandibular fossa
    B. Articular tubercle
    C. Condyle

Exercise 5: Evaluating Radiographs of Facial Bones

1. The mandibular rami are not superimposed, and the orbital roofs are not superimposed.
2. a. Fig. 21-26
   b. Fig. 21-24
   c. Fig. 21-25
3. a. The zygomatic arches are not symmetric, and the left zygomatic arch is superimposed with cranial structures.
   b. The midsagittal plane was not perpendicular to the cassette because the patient's head was slightly tilted.
4. a. The base of the occipital partially superimposes the mandible, and the mandibular rami are not seen without superimposition from surrounding structures.
   b. Reposition the head, ensuring that the forehead is in contact with the vertical grid device or x-ray table surface, to image the mandible without cranial superimposition.
5. a. The opposite side of the mandible superimposes the mandibular body.
   b. Position the head so that the uppermost side of the mandible will be projected above the mandibular body closer to the cassette.

Self-Test: Radiography of the Facial Bones

1. a	8. d	15. b
2. a	9. a	16. d
3. d	10. b	17. d
4. a	11. b	18. a
5. d	12. c	19. d
6. d	13. d	20. b
7. a	14. b	

CHAPTER 22 Paranasal Sinuses

Review

1. Frontal, sphenoidal, ethmoidal, and maxillary
2. A. Sphenoidal
   B. Maxillary
   C. Frontal
   D. Ethmoidal
3. a
4. b
5. d
6. d
7. c
8. c
9. To demonstrate the presence or absence of fluid and to differentiate between shadows caused by fluid and those caused by other pathologic conditions
10. Underpenetration produces shadows simulating pathologic conditions that do not exist.
11. a. Parallel
    b. Perpendicular
12. d
13. a
14. d
15. d
16. a, b, c, d, e, f
17. A. Frontal sinus
    B. Sella turcica
    C. Sphenoidal sinus
    D. Ethmoidal sinuses
    E. Maxillary sinus
    F. Superimposed mandibular rami
18. d
19. d
20. c
21. a
22. a
23. b
24. c, d, e, g, h, k, l, m
25. A. Frontal sinus
    B. Ethmoidal sinuses
    C. Petrous ridge
    D. Sphenoidal sinuses
    E. Maxillary sinus
26. Maxillary
27. Superimposed with the maxillary sinuses
28. Foreshortened
29. Orbitomeatal
30. Mentomeatal
31. Acanthion
32. Immediately below the maxillary sinuses
33. One on each side, just inferior to the medial aspect of the orbital floor and superior to the roof of the maxillary sinuses
34. False (Only the chin should touch the vertical grid device.)
35. True
36. c, e, g, j, k
37. A. Frontal sinus
    B. Ethmoidal sinuses
    C. Foramen rotundum
    D. Maxillary sinus
    E. Petrous pyramid
    F. Mastoid air cells
38. Acanthion
39. Chin
40. Orbitomeatal
41. Sphenoidal
42. c, e, g, h, j, k
43. False (The head should rest on its vertex.)
44. False (The infraorbitomeatal line should be as close to parallel with the cassette as possible.)
45. True
46. True
47. True
48. False (To demonstrate the paranasal sinuses, close restriction of the beam to the sinus area may exclude the occipital bone.)
49. Sphenoidal and ethmoidal
50. The mandibular symphysis should superimpose the anterior frontal bone.
51. Anterior to the petrous ridges
52. The infraorbitomeatal line was not parallel with the cassette because the neck was not extended far enough (assuming the central ray was correctly directed).
53. The infraorbitomeatal line was not parallel with the cassette because the neck was extended too far or the vertical cassette holder was tilted too far toward the patient (assuming the central ray was correctly directed).
54. d, e, f
55. A. Maxillary sinus
    B. Ethmoidal sinus
    C. Mandible
    D. Vomer
    E. Sphenoidal sinus
    F. Mandibular condyle
    G. Petrosa
56. True
57. True
58. False (Close beam restriction should be limited to the sinus area.)
59. False (Respiration should be suspended for the exposure.)
60. a
61. a. Perpendicular to the nasion
    b. 10 degrees cephalad to the glabella
    c. Perpendicular to a point midway between the infraorbital margins and acanthion
62. c
63. a
64. b
65. b, c, f

Self-Test: Radiography of the Paranasal Sinuses

1. d	8. a	14. d	20. a
2. a	9. a	15. b	21. b
3. d	10. b	16. c	22. c
4. d	11. d	17. d	23. d
5. b	12. c	18. c	24. c
6. a	13. d	19. a	25. b
7. b			

CHAPTER 23 **Temporal Bone**

Review

1. From true lateral, with the affected mastoid centered to the cassette, rotate the head until the midsagittal plane forms a 15-degree angle with the cassette.
2. a
3. c
4. d
5. 15 degrees caudad
6. Approximately 2 inches (5 cm) posterior and 2 inches (5 cm) above the uppermost external acoustic meatus
7. False (The head should be rotated 15 degrees from true lateral, moving the face closer to the cassette.)
8. False (The head should be rotated 15 degrees from true lateral, moving the face closer to the cassette.)
9. True
10. a, b, f, g, i, j
11. A. Internal and external acoustic meatus
    B. Mastoid air cells
    C. Mastoid process
    D. Mandibular condyle
12. Forehead, nose, and cheek
13. 12 degrees cephalad
14. d
15. d
16. d
17. c
18. A. Internal acoustic canal
    B. Arcuate eminence
    C. Mastoid air cells
    D. External acoustic meatus and canal
    E. Mandibular condyle
    F. Mastoid process
19. True
20. False (The midsagittal plane should form an angle of 45 degrees with the cassette.)
21. True
22. 10 degrees caudad
23. On the zygomatic bone approximately 1 inch (2.5 cm) anterior to and ¾ inch (2 cm) above the external acoustic meatus
24. d
25. b, e, f, g, h, j

Self-Test: Radiography of the Temporal Bone

1. d	6. c	11. b
2. d	7. a	12. c
3. d	8. d	13. b
4. d	9. d	14. b
5. c	10. a	15. a

CHAPTER 24 **Mammography**

SECTION 1 **Anatomy and Physiology of the Breast**

1. A. Axillary prolongation (tail) of the breast
   B. Serratus anterior
   C. Pectoralis minor
   D. Pectoralis major (cut)
2. A. Fat
   B. Nipple
   C. Lactiferous tubules
   D. Fat
   E. Inframammary crease
   F. Pectoralis major
   G. Retromammary fat
3. Milk
4. Mammary
5. Areola
6. 15; 20
7. Acini
8. Smaller
9. Involution
10. Fat
11. Lactiferous
12. Tail
13. Cooper's
14. Axilla
15. Sternum

SECTION 2 **Radiography of the Breast**

Exercise 1

1. Because the mammogram will record the slightest wrinkle in any cloth covering
2. These substances will resemble calcifications on the resultant image.
3. Craniocaudal and mediolateral oblique projections
4. To locate a nipple that is not in profile
5. Compress the breast with an approved mammographic compression device.
6. Place a radiopaque marker such as a BB on the breast overlying the mass.
7. To evaluate whether or not sufficient breast tissue is demonstrated
8. Nipple and chest wall, or edge of the image, whichever comes first
9. 1 cm
10. Clean the image receptor surface and face guard with a disinfectant.

Exercise 2

1. b
2. a, b, c, d
3. b, d
4. a, b, c
5. d
6. a, b, c, d
7. a
8. b
9. c
10. a

Self-Test: Mammography

1. a	6. d	11. b
2. c	7. a	12. a
3. d	8. c	13. c
4. c	9. c	14. c
5. b	10. d	15. a

CHAPTER 25 **Central Nervous System**

SECTION 1 **Anatomy of the Central Nervous System**

1. A. Cerebrum
   B. Corpus callosum
   C. Cerebrum
   D. Cerebellum
   E. Pituitary gland
   F. Medulla oblongata
   G. Cerebellum
   H. Pons
2. A. Gray substance
   B. White substance
   C. Posterior nerve root
   D. Anterior nerve root
3. A. Pons
   B. Medulla oblongata
   C. Spinal cord
   D. Dural sac for the cauda equina
4. A. Fourth ventricle
   B. Inferior horn
   C. Interventricular foramen
   D. Anterior horn
   E. Body of the lateral ventricle
   F. Third ventricle
   G. Posterior horn
   H. Cerebral aqueduct
5. A. Body of the lateral ventricle
   B. Anterior horn
   C. Inferior horn
6. A. Fourth ventricle
   B. Body of the lateral ventricle
   C. Third ventricle
   D. Anterior horn
   E. Inferior horn
   F. Lateral recess
   G. Posterior horn
7. Brain and spinal cord

8. Cerebrum, cerebellum, and brain stem
9. Diencephalon, midbrain (mesencephalon), pons, and medulla oblongata
10. Cerebellum, pons, and medulla oblongata
11. Cerebrum (forebrain)
12. Forebrain
13. Midbrain (mesencephalon)
14. Longitudinal fissure
15. Pituitary gland
16. Cerebellum
17. Medulla oblongata
18. Meninges
19. Pia mater
20. Dura mater
21. Lateral
22. Cerebrum (forebrain)
23. Interventricular
24. Monro
25. Cerebral aqueduct and aqueduct of Sylvius

SECTION 2 **Radiography of the Central Nervous System**

1. Radiographic examination of the spinal cord after the injection of a contrast medium into the subarachnoid space
2. L2-L3, L3-L4, and cisterna cerebellomedullaris (cisterna magna)
3. Extrinsic spinal cord compression
4. Nonionic, water-soluble (They provide good visualization of nerve roots and good enhancement for follow-up computerized tomography, and they are readily absorbed by the body.)
5. To prevent it from accidentally contacting the spinal needle
6. Explain details of the examination to the patient before beginning the procedure.
7. Prone and lateral recumbent with the spine flexed
8. Varying the angulation of the table
9. To compress the cisterna cerebellomedullaris, preventing the contrast medium from entering cranial structures
10. Cross-table lateral of the cervical spine

Self-Test: Central Nervous System

1. b	6. a	11. b
2. b	7. c	12. a
3. c	8. d	13. b
4. b	9. c	14. d
5. b	10. d	15. c

CHAPTER 26 **Circulatory System**

SECTION 1 **Anatomy of the Circulatory System**

Exercise 1

1. A. Superior sagittal sinus
   B. Transverse sinus
   C. Internal jugular vein
   D. Right subclavian artery and vein
   E. Superior vena cava
   F. Brachial artery and basilic vein
   G. Celiac axis (artery)
   H. Portal vein
   I. Renal artery and vein
   J. Superior mesenteric artery and vein
   K. Common iliac artery and vein
   L. Common femoral artery and vein
   M. Popliteal artery
   N. Anterior tibial artery
   O. Posterior tibial artery
   P. Anterior facial artery and vein
   Q. Common carotid artery
   R. Aortic arch
   S. Pulmonary artery and vein
   T. Aorta
   U. Inferior vena cava
   V. Inferior mesenteric vein
   W. Radial artery and cephalic vein
   X. Ulnar artery and basilic vein
   Y. Deep femoral artery
   Z. Superficial femoral artery
   AA. Popliteal vein
   BB. Large saphenous vein
2. A. Aortic arch
   B. Superior vena cava
   C. Right pulmonary artery
   D. Right pulmonary veins
   E. Right atrium
   F. Right atrioventricular (tricuspid) valve
   G. Right ventricle
   H. Inferior vena cava
   I. Descending aorta
   J. Left ventricle
   K. Left atrioventricular (bicuspid or mitral) valve
   L. Left lung
   M. Left atrium
3. A. Right coronary artery
   B. Left coronary artery
4. A. Coronary sinus
   B. Great cardiac vein

5. A. Capillaries
   B. Lungs
   C. Right atrium
   D. Right ventricle
   E. Liver
   F. Intestine
   G. Aorta
   H. Left atrium
   I. Left ventricle
   J. Stomach
   K. Spleen
   L. Pancreas
6. A. External carotid artery
   B. Internal carotid artery
   C. Right common carotid artery
   D. Right vertebral artery
   E. Right subclavian artery
   F. Brachiocephalic artery
   G. Brachial artery
   H. Radial artery
   I. Ulnar artery
   J. Left subclavian artery
   K. Left vertebral artery
   L. Left common carotid artery
   M. Thyroid
7. A. Axillary nodes
   B. Common iliac nodes
   C. Deep inguinal nodes
   D. Cervical nodes
   E. Thoracic duct
   F. Lumbar nodes
   G. Superior inguinal nodes

Exercise 2

1. Blood-vascular; lymphatic
2. Pulmonary; systemic
3. Pulmonary
4. Arteries
5. Veins
6. Arterioles
7. Capillaries
8. Venules
9. Venules
10. Pulmonary
11. Superior vena cava
12. Inferior vena cava
13. Myocardium
14. Endocardium
15. Epicardium
16. Left ventricle
17. Pericardial cavity
18. Atria
19. Ventricles
20. Atria
21. Ventricles
22. Tricuspid
23. Mitral; bicuspid
24. Right
25. Left
26. Left ventricle

27. Coronary
28. Cardiac
29. Right
30. Aorta
31. Iliac
32. Femoral
33. Popliteal
34. Tibial
35. Portal
36. Hepatic
37. Inferior vena cava
38. Pulmonary
39. Pulmonary
40. Pulmonary
41. Systole
42. Diastole
43. Common carotid; vertebral
44. Left common carotid
45. Subclavian
46. Basilar
47. Internal; external
48. Cerebral
49. Posterior cerebral
50. Jugular
51. Brachiocephalic
52. Subclavian
53. Brachial
54. Radial; ulnar
55. Forearm
56. Aorta (abdominal)
57. Brain
58. Heart
59. Thoracic
60. Subclavian; jugular

SECTION 2 **Radiography of the Circulatory System**

1. The risk of extravasation is reduced; most body parts can be reached for selective injection; the patient can be positioned as needed; and the catheter can be safely left in the body while the radiographs are being examined.
2. Seldinger
3. Femoral
4. b
5. b, c, g
6. b, d, e
7. The patient's legs should be elevated and intravenous fluids may be administered.
8. To reduce the possibility of the aspiration of vomitus
9. To saturate the kidneys and minimize kidney damage from iodinated contrast media
10. T6

11. A. Brachiocephalic artery
    B. Ascending aorta
    C. Right coronary artery
    D. Intercostal arteries
    E. Left common carotid artery
    F. Left subclavian artery
    G. Left coronary artery
    H. Descending thoracic aorta
12. From the diaphragm to the aortic bifurcation
13. Lateral
14. A. Hepatic artery
    B. Right renal artery
    C. Right common iliac artery
    D. Splenic artery
    E. Left renal artery
    F. Abdominal aorta
15. A. Celiac axis
    B. Superior mesenteric artery
    C. Abdominal aorta
16. AP
17. Expiration
18. A. Left gastric artery
    B. Hepatic artery
    C. Gastroduodenal artery
    D. Splenic artery
    E. Celiac axis
19. To ensure exact positioning of the tube-part-film alignment and close collimation of the x-ray tube
20. Splenic
21. Proximally
22. Upper
23. a
24. b
25. b
26. A. Ulnar artery
    B. Posterior interosseous artery
    C. Brachial artery
    D. Right subclavian artery
27. In the superficial vein at the wrist (when demonstrating the entire upper limb) or at the elbow (when demonstrating the upper arm)
28. A. Cephalic vein
    B. Basilic vein
    C. Subclavian vein
29. Extended and internally rotated 30 degrees
30. A. Common iliac artery
    B. External iliac artery
    C. Profunda femoris artery
    D. Femoral artery
    E. Popliteal artery
    F. Anterior tibial artery
    G. Peroneal artery
    H. Posterior tibial artery
31. c
32. c
33. a
34. c
35. a

36. a. Capillary
    b. Arterial
    c. Venous
37. Infraorbitomeatal
38. Away from the injected side
39. a
40. b

Self-Test: Anatomy and Radiography of the Circulatory System

1. c	6. b	11. c	16. d
2. d	7. a	12. b	17. b
3. c	8. a	13. c	18. a
4. a	9. a	14. c	19. b
5. d	10. b	15. c	20. d

CHAPTER 27 Sectional Anatomy for Radiographers

Review

1. A. Frontal bone
   B. Superior sagittal sinus
   C. Parietal bone
   D. White matter
   E. Falx cerebri (longitudinal fissure)
2. A. Genu of the corpus callosum
   B. Internal capsule
   C. Basal nuclei
   D. Third ventricle
   E. Occipital lobe
   F. Longitudinal fissure
   G. Anterior horn of the lateral ventricle
   H. Caudate nucleus
   I. Thalamus
   J. Posterior horn of the lateral ventricle
3. A. Longitudinal fissure
   B. Middle cerebral artery
   C. Basilar artery
   D. Pons
   E. Fourth ventricle
   F. Cerebellum
   G. Frontal lobe
   H. Frontal sinus
   I. Anterior cerebral artery
   J. Posterior cerebral artery
   K. Mastoid air cells
4. A. Sphenoidal sinus
   B. Internal carotid artery
   C. Pars petrosa
   D. Auricle of the ear
   E. Ethmoidal sinuses
   F. Ocular bulb
   G. Optic nerve
   H. Temporal lobe
   I. Basilar artery
   J. Pons
   K. Cerebellum

5. A. Mandibular symphysis
   B. Hyoid
   C. Submandibular gland
   D. Common carotid artery
   E. Sternocleidomastoid muscle
   F. Internal jugular vein
   G. Epiglottic cartilage
   H. Laryngeal pharynx
6. A. Common carotid artery
   B. Thyroid gland
   C. Thyroid cartilage
   D. Larynx
   E. Pharynx
   F. Internal jugular vein
   G. Trapezius muscle
   H. Body of the T6 vertebra
   I. Vertebral artery
7. A. Lateral ventricle
   B. Third ventricle
   C. Optic chiasm
   D. Pituitary gland
   E. Sphenoidal sinus
   F. Clivus
   G. Nasopharynx
   H. Maxilla
   I. Tongue
   J. Corpus callosum
   K. Great cerebral vein (of Galen)
   L. Corpora quadrigemina
   M. Cerebral aqueduct
   N. Straight sinus
   O. Cerebellum
   P. Fourth ventricle
   Q. Pons
   R. Basilar artery
   S. Cervical spinal cord
   T. C2 vertebra
8. A. Superior sagittal sinus
   B. Longitudinal fissure
   C. Corpus callosum
   D. Lateral ventricle
   E. Septum pellucidum
   F. Lateral fissure
   G. Sphenoidal sinus
   H. Mandibular ramus
   I. Masseter muscle
   J. Submandibular gland
   K. Caudate nucleus
   L. Basal nuclei
   M. Third ventricle
   N. Optic chiasm
   O. Pituitary gland
   P. Internal carotid artery
   Q. Nasopharynx
   R. Medial pterygoid muscle
   S. Oropharynx

9. A. Superior sagittal sinus
   B. Lateral ventricle
   C. Third ventricle
   D. External acoustic canal
   E. Parotid gland
   F. Dens
   G. Vertebral artery
   H. Internal carotid artery
   I. Thalamus
   J. Cranial nerves (in the internal acoustic canal)
   K. Sternocleidomastoid muscle
10. A. Lateral ventricle
    B. Pineal body
    C. Superior and inferior colliculi
    D. Auricle
    E. Middle cerebellar peduncle
    F. Medulla oblongata
    G. Cervical spinal cord
    H. Corpus callosum (splenium)
    I. Cerebral aqueduct
    J. Cerebellum
    K. Mastoid region
11. A. Manubrium
    B. Brachiocephalic artery
    C. Right brachiocephalic vein
    D. Trachea
    E. Esophagus
    F. Scapula
    G. Left common carotid artery
    H. Left brachiocephalic vein
    I. Left subclavian artery
    J. Left lung
12. A. Sternum
    B. Ascending aorta
    C. Superior vena cava
    D. Right pulmonary artery
    E. Right primary bronchus
    F. Azygos vein
    G. Body of the T5 vertebra
    H. Pulmonary trunk
    I. Left pulmonary artery
    J. Descending aorta
    K. Scapula
13. A. Serratus anterior muscle
    B. Liver
    C. Right atrium
    D. Right ventricle
    E. Sternum
    F. Left ventricle
    G. Esophagus
    H. Latissimus dorsi muscle
    I. Descending aorta
    J. Azygos vein
    K. Inferior vena cava

14. A. Pharynx
    B. Tongue
    C. Epiglottis
    D. Trachea
    E. Left brachiocephalic vein
    F. Manubrium
    G. C2 vertebra
    H. Spinal cord
    I. Intervertebral disk
    J. Brachiocephalic artery
    K. Aortic arch
    L. Right pulmonary artery
15. A. Spinal cord
    B. Sternocleidomastoid muscle
    C. Right lung
    D. Tracheal bifurcation
    E. Heart
    F. Left subclavian artery
    G. Clavicle
    H. Acromion
    I. Humeral head
    J. Aortic arch
    K. Pulmonary trunk
16. A. Liver
    B. Lower lobe of the right lung
    C. Stomach
    D. Diaphragm
    E. Spleen
    F. Esophagus
    G. Aorta
17. A. Caudate lobe
    B. Right lobe of the liver
    C. Portal vein
    D. Quadrate lobe
    E. Ligamentum teres
    F. Left lobe of the liver
    G. Stomach
    H. Aorta
    I. Spleen
    J. Crus of the diaphragm
    K. Inferior vena cava
18. A. Superior mesenteric artery
    B. Right lobe of the liver
    C. Inferior vena cava
    D. Right kidney
    E. Crus of the diaphragm
    F. Stomach
    G. Rectus abdominis muscle
    H. Body of the pancreas
    I. Left colic flexure
    J. Aorta
19. A. Inferior vena cava
    B. Right lobe of the liver
    C. Aorta
    D. Left kidney
    E. Stomach (with contrast)
    F. Tail of the pancreas
    G. Spleen

20. A. Psoas major muscle
    B. Iliacus (iliac) muscle
    C. Ureter
    D. Rectus abdominis muscle
    E. Anterior superior iliac spine (ASIS)
    F. Ilium
    G. Sacroiliac (SI) joint
21. A. Femoral vessels
    B. Pubic symphysis
    C. Bladder
    D. Acetabulum
    E. Head of the femur
    F. Rectum
    G. Gluteus
22. A. Obturator externus muscle
    B. Obturator internus muscle
    C. Greater trochanter
    D. Prostate
    E. Rectum
    F. Spermatic cord
    G. Corpora cavernosa (of the penis)
    H. Pubic bone
    I. Femoral vessels
    J. Femoral head
    K. Gluteus maximus muscle
    L. Ischium
23. A. Aorta
    B. Rectus abdominis muscle
    C. Bladder
    D. Pubic bone
    E. Corpora cavernosa
    F. Cauda equina
    G. L4 vertebra
    H. Sacrum
    I. Rectum
    J. Coccyx
    K. Prostatic urethra (within the prostate)
    L. Corpus spongiosum
    M. Testicles (testes)
24. A. Sigmoid colon
    B. Bladder
    C. Ductus deferens
    D. Prostate
    E. Gracilis muscle
    F. Psoas muscle
    G. Iliacus (iliac) muscle
    H. Ilium
    I. Gluteus medius muscle
    J. Gluteus minimus muscle
    K. Acetabulum
    L. Pubic ramus
    M. Corpus spongiosum
    N. Scrotum

APPENDIX Supplemental Exercises for Skull Positioning

Skull Positioning Review

Exercise 1

1. o
2. n
3. p
4. n
5. c
6. m
7. a
8. f
9. m
10. f
11. b
12. e
13. a
14. a
15. f

Exercise 2

1. n
2. f
3. d
4. o
5. i
6. j
7. g
8. a
9. c
10. b
11. h
12. k
13. p
14. l
15. m

Exercise 3

1. H
2. N
3. A
4. D
5. J
6. K
7. I
8. F
9. G
10. R
11. H
12. O

13. H
14. S
15. P
16. Q
17. H
18. K
19. M

20. E
21. M
22. B
23. C
24. O
25. S